AF615851

PSYCHIATRY: COMMON DRUG TREATMENTS

PRACTICAL PROBLEMS IN MEDICINE

Psychiatry: Common Drug Treatments

Roy Spector, FRCP, FRCPath
Professor of Applied Pharmacology, Guy's Hospital Medical School

Howard Rogers, MA, PhD, MRCP, MRCS
Reader in Clinical Pharmacology, Guy's Hospital Medical School, and Consultant Physician, Guy's Hospital

David Roy, MB, MRCPsych
Consultant Psychiatrist, Goodmayes Hospital, and Senior Lecturer in Psychiatry, St Bartholomew's Hospital

Series Consultant
John Fry, OBE, MD, FRCS, FRCGP

MARTIN DUNITZ

First published in the United Kingdom in 1984
by Martin Dunitz Limited, London

British Library Cataloguing in Publication Data

Spector, R. G.
Psychiatry.—(Practical problems in medicine)
1. Psychopharmacology
I. Title II. Rogers, H. J.
III. Roy, David J. IV. Series
616.89'18 RC483

ISBN 0-906348-64-1

Designed and phototypeset by BookEns,
Saffron Walden, Essex
Printed and bound in Singapore by
Toppan Printing Company (S) Pte Ltd

Drug trade names

Throughout the text, most drugs are referred to by their generic names only. A table of British and Australian trade names has been included in the appendix.

Contents

List of illustrations

Acknowledgements

The authors are very grateful to Dr Paul Bridges, Department of Psychiatry, Guy's Hospital.

The publishers are grateful to David Gifford for drawing the diagrams and to Jennifer Eaton, MSc, MPS, for information on international drug-name equivalents. The table on page 119 was prepared using research material from the Metropolitan Life Insurance Co., New York.

1
Psychiatric aspects of medicine

BACKGROUND

The psychiatric aspects of medicine occupy a uniquely important place in clinical practice. This is not only because, numerically, psychiatric illness makes a major contribution to hospital bed occupancy, to consultations in hospital practice and general practice, and to the State's drug bill, but particularly because of the nature of the disturbances produced. Mental illness involves the most precious of human attributes such as creativity, imagination, love, humour, ability to identify with others and the wish to build up and sustain family life. These essentially human qualities are often the most vulnerable to disease processes.

Compared with our understanding of physical illness – such as mitral stenosis or impetigo – we know little about the nature of mental illness. There is as yet no pathology of these conditions. At present hypotheses are being developed, but we are even uncertain as to the appropriateness of our language of psychopathology. Computer models of brain function are not yet advanced enough even to address the problem of the relationship of mind and brain. However, even though our theories prove inadequate for the total problem, if they can make predictions that will direct one or two useful steps forward, then they can be considered respectable scientifically.

But psychiatry is not only concerned with the higher flights of human subtleties. Some mental illness is devastating and destructive. Schizophrenia, for example, is the most malign of all non-fatal diseases. Patients who have suffered severe physical and mental illness have compared the pain of depression with that of terminal cancer. There are not many physical illnesses which drive the sufferer to suicide.

The importance of psychiatry is further enhanced by the fact that psychological factors frequently compound primarily physical problems. The pain of a prolapsed intervertebral disc, for example, produces apprehension and consequent muscular tension and spasm which augment the initial painful lesion.

PSYCHOTROPIC DRUGS

Initial trials

Up to the mid-1950s no specific psychotropic drugs were available – apart from hypnosedatives and the amphetamine type of stimulants. Around that time chlorpromazine, the monoamine oxidase inhibitors and the tricyclic antidepressants were introduced in rapid succession. These had a great impact on medical practice. Schizophrenic patients were no longer condemned to a life in a mental hospital, the victims of insulting and terrifying voices and delusions of persecution. The introduction of chlorpromazine meant that there was no longer a need to build long-stay psychiatric hospitals, nor to make straightjackets and padded cells. In humanitarian and historical terms the importance of the discovery of this single drug cannot be overstated.

Recent trends

Since the 1950s a continuous stream of powerful and varied psychotropic drugs has become available to medical practitioners. In conjunction with the great need for such agents all seemed set for a happy marriage. However, there are problems with the psychotropic drugs. They are not without toxic effects and fortunately they do not alter the personality and social setting of the patient. Thus their actions are frequently incomplete or transient, and yet prolonged or more intense drug treatment may lead to dependence or toxicity. The art seems to be to know when to use the drugs – and, even more importantly, when to stop.

Drugs and the patient

In many mental illnesses, symptoms arise because of an interaction between a vulnerable personality and a stressful environment. Even the most resilient person will become ill if life events become sufficiently difficult. The first important therapeutic step is to listen with the greatest possible concentration to the patient. This may not only lead to the understanding of the nature of the individual's personality and his environment, but listening in itself is powerful therapy. To be listened to is to be esteemed. As in general medicine, the patient presenting with psychological symptoms should come to understand the nature of his condition. He should, where possible, also be party to the decision to use a particular method of treatment. If drugs are to be used he must clearly understand the dosage scheme and how long the treatment is to last. The patient, even during a course of drug therapy does not have to be passive. In the treatment of phobias and anxiety states, for example, a short course of anxiolytic agents may be an opportunity for the patient to expose himself (and thus produce desensitization) to situations which had been fear-provoking. Possible toxicity of drugs should be discussed with the patient in such a way as not to cause alarm.

Classification

Although several methods of classifying drugs used in mental illness exist, the most useful of these from a clinical point of view groups the drugs according to their principal actions and indications. One such classification is:

- Neuroleptics
- Anxiolytic – sedatives
- Antidepressants
- Mood stabilizers
- Stimulants
- Hallucinogens

The use of stimulants (such as amphetamine) is limited and only rarely used by general physicians. Hallucinogens are even less commonly used – and at best their clinical applications are debatable. However, the field is rapidly changing. In recent months some synthetic cannabinoids – particularly nabilone – have been used in terminal illness as antiemetics, sedatives and analgesics.

EPIDEMIOLOGY AND NATURAL HISTORY

The magnitude of the problems posed by mental illness can be assessed by examining the incidence of some of the conditions. About 10–20 per cent of consultations in general practice are related to neurotic illness – most frequently anxiety and reactive depression. Almost every individual in a lifetime will suffer from fear, tension or apprehension out of proportion to the size of the threat which precipitated the reaction. One-third of the population consults a doctor because of such neurotic reactions.

Endogenous depression often occurs in repeated, self-limiting attacks. The condition is severe enough to necessitate referral to a specialist in 8 per 1000 of the population. Of all types of depression, an average of 30 new cases a year are seen in a general medical practice of 3000 patients. In some surveys about one-quarter of married women with young children suffer from depression – usually of the neurotic (or reactive type).

Schizophrenia is the most severe of all non-killing diseases and has an incidence in the general population of approximately 8 per 1000. About one-half of schizophrenics previously showed a premorbid 'schizoid' personality, consisting of detachment, secretiveness, emotional coolness, shyness and seclusiveness. Slow onset and intellectual deterioration are associated with a poor prognosis, but favourable features are an acute onset of symptoms and a clear external trigger crisis at the onset. After a single hospital admission 50 per cent of patients do not relapse, but after more than one admission only 20 per cent are free of symptoms five years after the initial diagnosis.

PRACTICAL POINTS

- The importance of psychiatry in medicine is enhanced by the fact that psychological factors frequently compound basically physical problems.
- The introduction of the drug chlorpromazine has had more effect on the treatment of schizophrenia than any other comparable drug.
- Psychotropic drugs are not without toxic side-effects so it is vital to know when to use, and when to stop using, these drugs.
- Patients should be fully consulted about all aspects of their drug treatment.
- Endogenous depression is a severe enough condition to necessitate referral to a specialist in 8 per 1000 of the population.

2
Neuroleptic drugs

BACKGROUND

Neuroleptic drugs, particularly chlorpromazine, are mainly used in the treatment of schizophrenia, but they are also used in acute organic psychoses, paranoid psychoses, or alcohol withdrawal. This chapter deals mainly with the neuroleptic drugs and their effects in the treatment of schizophrenic states.

RECOGNIZING, DIAGNOSING AND TREATING SCHIZOPHRENIA

The word 'schizophrenia' was first introduced by Eugen Bleuler in 1911[1]. In lay terminology it is commonly misinterpreted as 'split-personality', a problem which has little to do with schizophrenia.

The traditional classifications of schizophrenia are hebephrenic, catatonic, paranoid and simple. It may be more useful to think of these in descriptive rather than diagnostic terms in view of considerable overlap of symptoms.

Hebephrenic schizophrenia

The hebephrenic patient is young, emotionally inappropriate and thought-disordered.

Catatonic schizophrenia

This describes the illness with motor disorders and occasional stupor. It is now less common than it used to be – possibly due to treatment starting much earlier.

Paranoid schizophrenia

Paranoid schizophrenics are often older and experience persecutory delusions, usually having a more intact personality with warm affective responses.

Simple schizophrenia

In this condition the patient is typically a young adult with poor social interactions, loss of motivation and flattening of affect. In this form the illness has a relentlessly progressive course.

Nuclear schizophrenia

A diagnosis of schizophrenia which has the features of early and insidious onset with a seemingly relentless course is now often called nuclear.

Symptoms and diagnosis

The symptoms which have been identified as diagnostic of schizophrenia are called first-rank symptoms and were described by Schneider in 1959. They consist of:

- Auditory hallucinations (often in the form of a running commentary)
- Audible thoughts (*Gedankenlautwerden*)
- Thought withdrawal, insertion and interruption
- Thought broadcast
- Delusional perceptions
- External control of emotions
- Somatic passivity and feelings, drives or acts due to the influence of others

These should be considered diagnostic only when taken in association with family history, type of onset, age and premorbid personality.

Drug treatment

It is common practice that a psychotic patient is treated with neuroleptic medication immediately on admission to hospital or even in the outpatients' clinic. Unnecessary delay in treatment has been associated with poorer prognosis, but overhasty treatment in diagnostically doubtful cases is equally unhelpful. Most schizophrenic patients are diagnosed and established on medication in hospital. Some patients follow a chronic course with few acute episodes and remain fairly stable on maintenance medication. Others show a progressive deterioration punctuated by frequent acute episodes, even when taking high doses of a neuroleptic drug.

There is a trend among psychiatrists to delay before making a diagnosis of schizophrenia. Thus acute psychotic episodes with schizophrenic features which respond to medication and never relapse may not be diagnosed as schizophrenia at all. In this group maintenance medication is usually withdrawn early.

Schizophrenics are poor at taking tablets and the compliance is well below 50 per cent; however, with the introduction of the injectable depot neuroleptics (see page 25), the relapse rate in schizophrenics has diminished.

There have been a number of studies conducted whereby the depot injection has been replaced with placebo and there has been a significant increase in acute relapse rate. Because of this, depot injections have become the mainstay in treatment of the schizophrenic patient.

In the majority of patients the drug treatment of schizophrenia itself is confined to the neuroleptics. Antidepressants, particularly the tricyclics, can occasionally cause an exacerbation of psychotic symptoms. Depressive symptoms, however, are common in schizophrenia and, when severe, antidepressant medication may be required. Many

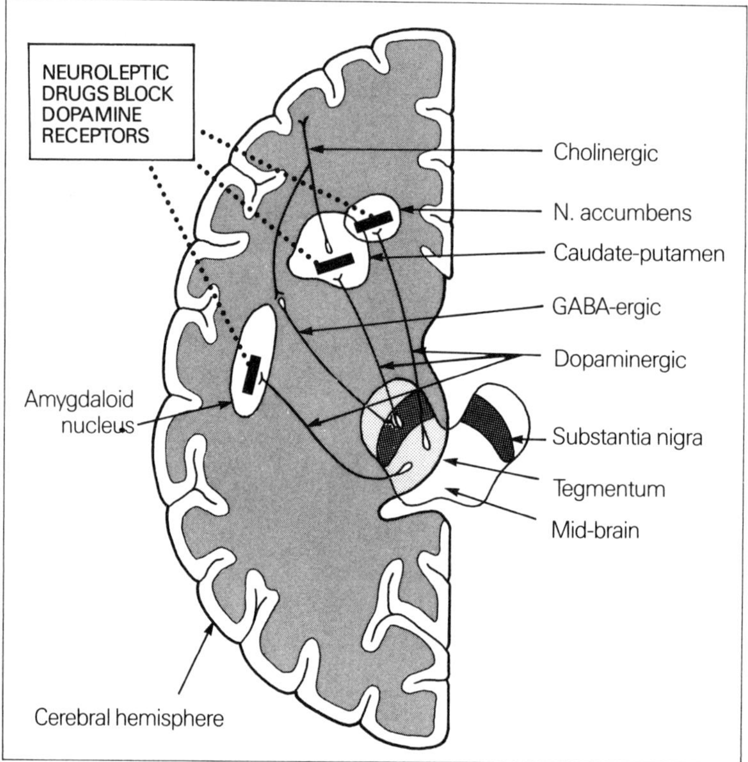

Figure 1 Diagrammatical section of a cerebral hemisphere showing three dopaminergic pathways – all of which are blocked by neuroleptics. Interference with the nigrostriatal pathway (substantia nigra to caudate) results in parkinsonism. Blockade of the pathways between the tegmentum, amygdala and nucleus accumbens causes emotional indifference and may be responsible for the antipsychotic effects of these drugs.

schizophrenic patients develop symptoms identified as depressive as a part of an acute relapse of the schizophrenic illness itself, and remission of those symptoms corresponds with successful management of the schizophrenia.

Hypnotic medication in the form of benzodiazepines is commonly prescribed. Sleep disturbance is sometimes a troublesome feature of a schizophrenic breakdown, and the same guidlines apply as for all secondary insomnia problems, namely that the successful treatment of the underlying problem should result in the resolution of the sleep disturbance (see Chapter 6).

CLASSIFICATION AND EFFECTS OF NEUROLEPTICS

The neuroleptics available range from those with potent dopamine blocking activity and mild sedative potential, to those with less severe dopamine blockade and subsequently slightly less severe extrapyramidal side-effects (see page 26), but more sedative action.

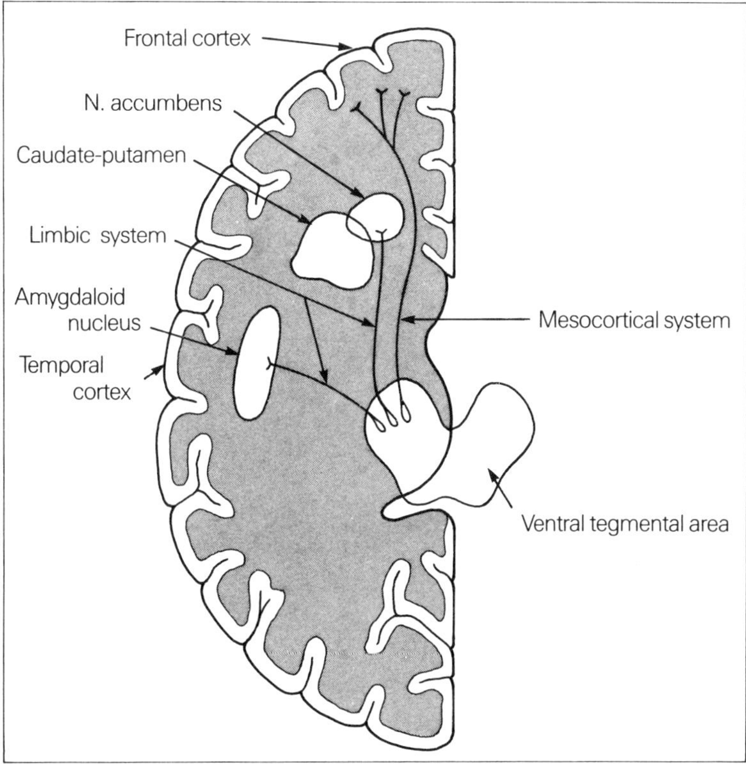

Figure 2 Diagrammatical horizontal section of cerebral hemisphere and mid-brain showing part of the limbic system and mesocortical systems. Both sets of pathways are concerned with the expression, integration and memory of emotional reactions.

Chlorpromazine has both moderate sedative properties and extrapyramidal side-effects and is the most widely prescribed neuroleptic. The most commonly prescribed of the less sedative drugs are haloperidol and pimozide. The more sedative drugs are thioridazine and promazine.

Drugs with less extrapyramidal side-effects may prove particularly useful in the elderly where these side-effects and other movement disorders may occur up to eight times more frequently than in the young. While sedation might be a serious problem, long-term movement disorders might well be minimized by using thioridazine or promazine in this age group.

Dopamine and drug action

The introduction of chlorpromazine in 1952 for the treatment of excited psychotic states dramatically affected the drug treatment of schizophrenia. Since then other drugs have been developed which are also effective in this illness. Although many of the antipsychotic drugs bear little structural resemblance to other members of the group, they all share a common effect – to antagonize the actions of dopamine. One implication of such an unexpected finding is that schizophrenia may have a biochemical basis involving excessive dopaminergic activity. Dopamine is a normal constituent of the brain and is one of the amine neurotransmitters. When dopamine activity is artificially increased in the nervous system (as by administration of amphetamine or levodopa) psychotic reactions, including hallucinations and paranoia, can result.

Mesolimbic formation This is concerned with the integration of emotional responses and possibly with the memory of emotionally charged experiences. Dopamine is a neurotransmitter in this system, but it is also a transmitter in other regions, such as the chemoreceptor trigger zone and the extrapyramidal system. With hindsight it does not seem surprising that the antipsychotic drugs act on these parts of the brain. The majority are powerfully antiemetic and can produce parkinsonism and other extrapyramidal disturbances. These drugs, which have been called major tranquillizers, are now referred to as neuroleptics; they include the following groups of drugs:

- Phenothiazines
- Butyrophenones
- Thioxanthines
- Diphenylbutylpiperidines
- Dihydroindoles
- Dibenzodiazepines

PHENOTHIAZINES

Although the neuroleptics in this group possess the basic tricyclic phenothiazine nucleus, they may be divided into three subcategories according to the type of side-chain attached to the ring nitrogen atom. This influences some of the side-effects.

Subcategories of phenothiazines

Side-chain	Sedation	Atropine-like actions	Parkinsonism and antiemetic activity	Alpha-blockade and hypotension
Aliphatic	Moderate	Moderate	Moderate	Moderate
Piperidine	Much	Much	Little	Much
Piperazine	Little	Little	Much	Little

Actions and side-effects

1. All the drugs in the above table possess antipsychotic and antihallucinatory properties.
2. Large doses are usually sedating, but with smaller doses the patients are

Phenothiazines with neuroleptic activity, possessing the types of side-chain shown in the table opposite

Drug	Dose	Special features
Aliphatic side-chain		
Chlorpromazine	100–2000 mg orally daily (divided doses) Also intramuscularly and intravenously 25–100 mg. 100 mg per rectum	Antiemetic, antihiccough; also useful in excited organic states (including narcotic withdrawal) and in the elderly; not recommended for alcohol or barbiturate dependence because it can aggravate fits
Promazine	100–400 mg orally daily (divided doses) Also intramuscularly 50 mg	Useful in senile agitation
Piperidine side-chain		
Thioridazine	100–800 mg orally daily (divided doses)	Useful sedative in the elderly with little extrapyramidal effects; little antiemetic activity; can produce postural fainting
Piperazine side-chain		
Trifluoperazine	2–6 mg orally daily (divided doses) 1–3 mg intramuscularly daily	Powerful antiemetic Used in some dyskinesias
Prochlorperazine	5–50 mg orally daily (divided doses) 1–2 ml intramuscularly of 1.25 per cent solution of mesylate 5–25 mg per rectum	Powerful antiemetic: may be helpful in Ménière's disease
Thiopropazate	10–30 mg orally daily (divided doses)	May cause severe dermatitis when handled repeatedly; used in chorea.
Perphenazine	6–30 mg orally daily (divided doses)	Antiemetic
Fluphenazine	Fluphenazine hydrochloride 1–10 mg orally and intramuscularly daily Fluphenazine decanoate 12.5–2.5 mg intramuscularly every 2–4 weeks	Long-acting depot neuroleptic

quiet and unresponsive because there is emotional indifference to inner and external events. This emotional flatness is called the ataractic state and can constitute a severe social disability when these drugs are used for long periods.

3. Due to inhibitory actions on the brain-stem autonomic nuclei, chemoreceptor trigger zone and hypothalamus the drugs are hypotensive, antiemetic and antihiccough. Other consequences of hypothalamic inhibition are hypothermia and increased prolactin release.
4. A range of extrapyramidal toxic effects can develop, but pre-existing chorea can be diminished.
5. Pre-existing epilepsy can be aggravated (particularly in alcoholics).
6. Sex dysfunction – such as impotence, galactorrhoea and amenorrhoea – are due to hyperprolactinaemia (see Chapter 9).
7. All the above are due to actions on the brain. In addition peripheral effects are produced:
   - Alpha-adrenoceptor blockade (which contributes to postural hypotension, fainting and ejaculatory failure)
   - Powerful anticholinergic
   - Weak quinidine-like action on heart
   - Local anaesthetic
   - Weak antihistamine (H_1).

Toxic effects

1. Those mentioned in the previous section on basic actions, for example, fits, postural hypotension, anticholinergic (retention of urine, constipation, dry mouth, blurred vision, aggravation of glaucoma), sedation, depression, emotional inertia, extrapyramidal toxicity (parkinsonism, tremor, bradykinesia, dystonia, akathisia, tardive dyskinesia – see also page 26).
2. Cholestatic jaundice.
3. Corneal and lens opacities, pigmentary retinopathy.
4. Light sensitivity dermatitis and pigmentation; urticaria.
5. Cardiac arrhythmias, cardiac arrest.
6. Leucopenia, thrombocytopenia (both rare).
7. Raised low-density lipoprotein (LDL) cholesterol, impaired glucose tolerance, amenorrhoea, gynaecomastia, galactorrhoea.
8. Potentiation of: sedation due to alcohol and anxiolytics; hypotensive drugs; anticholinergic drugs.

Chlorpromazine

Development This drug was developed from promethazine. The latter was synthesized in the 1930s and was found to have powerful antihistamine and sedative properties. Up to 1950 several trials of promethazine were carried out in an attempt to treat excited psychotic patients. These were unsuccessful, but in 1952 the French surgeon Laborit published his work on sedation in surgical practice[2]. He and his co-workers found that promethazine increased the actions of anaesthetic agents. In a search for other anaesthesia-potentiating agents chlorpromazine was synthesized. An important modification in the structure was lengthening the side-chain of the phenothiazine nucleus from two carbons (in promethazine) to three carbons (in chlorpromazine). Laborit tested the new compound and found not only prolongation of anaesthesia but also a global reduction in autonomic activity with cooling. This he describes as 'artificial hibernation' and was accompanied by a reduction in interest in what was going on around the subject. These actions were called ataractic or neuroleptic.

In 1951 and 1952 a number of physicians in France first observed the effectiveness of chlorpromazine in mania, paranoia and agitation and anxiety. The drug was released for general use in 1954 and in the same year H. E. Lehman and G. E. Hanrahan published in the *Archives of Neurology and Psychiatry* convincing evidence that chlorpromazine was remarkably effective in the treatment of psychomotor excitement and mania[3]. Although it was found to have a large number of other actions (hence the trade name Largactil) – such as antiemetic, antihiccough, antishivering, hypotensive and muscle-relaxant effects – its main use became established in the treatment of schizophrenia.

Up to that time there was no effective drug treatment for this terrible disease. Approximately 80 per cent of patients were in long-term hospital accommodation five years after diagnosis. Before 1954, straightjackets and padded cells were used to restrain and protect schizophrenic patients; with the introduction of chlorpromazine the need for mechanical restraint declined dramatically. The historical importance of this discovery cannot be overstated. For the first time it was possible to terminate acute schizophrenic episodes, arrest the progress of the disease and even to improve the mental state of patients who had previously been in mental hospitals for many years. Chronic schizophrenia was not eliminated, but patients who previously could not live outside hospital could, with chlorpromazine treatment, return home and carry out work – albeit in most instances in sheltered workshops.

Pharmacokinetics Chlorpromazine is absorbed following oral and intramuscular administration. However, the bioavailability of a single oral dose is only about 30 per cent of that of an intramuscular injection. First-pass metabolism in the intestinal wall has been thought to contribute to the low bioavailability of the drug taken by mouth, but hepatic metabolism plays a most important role. Estimates of the elimination half-life ($t_{1/2}\beta$) vary between 4 and 42 hours. The existence of an even deeper compartment for chlorpromazine and its metabolites seems likely, since after discontinuation of the drug in chronically treated patients, metabolites and even free chlorpromazine can be detected in the urine for 6–18 months. The elimination phase is preceded by an initial distribution (α) phase with a half-life of 3 hours. Both the α and β half-lives are not prolonged in patients suffering from cirrhosis. In different individuals the volume of distribution of chlorpromazine varies between 32 and 150 l/kg. The drug is highly tissue bound and 98–99 per cent bound to plasma proteins. It penetrates the blood–brain barrier and there is a good correlation between unbound plasma and cerebrospinal fluid (CSF) levels.

Not all patients with schizophrenia respond to chlorpromazine. One possible reason for this is that adequate tissue levels of the drug are not always attained. On fixed dose regimes tenfold interindividual and intraindividual variations in plasma level occur. Chlorpromazine is extensively metabolized along many pathways; 168 metabolites have been described and a large number of these have been detected in human urine following chlorpromazine administration. Some of the principal metabolites are:

- Chlorpromazine sulphoxide (CPZ-SO)
- 7-hydroxychlorpromazine and its glucuronide (7OH-CPZ)
- 7-hydroxy nor_1 and nor_2 chlorpromazine and their glucoronides.

There is no consensus of opinion relating plasma levels of chlorpromazine with therapeutic response in psychotic patients although there are good correlations between blood levels and autonomic changes and drowsiness. Because chlorpromazine has so many metabolites, only a few of which have yet been studied in relation to clinical response, it will therefore be difficult to show a positive relationship between only a fraction of the total drug and/or active metabolites and clinical effects.

Chronic administration of neuroleptics leads to tolerance of some of the side-effects. Because of dopamine blockade in the hypothalamus, chlorpromazine causes increased secretion of prolactin. However, no correlation is found between plasma chlorpromazine levels, prolactin levels and extrapyramidal side-effects in patients on chronic treatment, although this correlation holds in patients treated for short periods. Since the plasma blood levels are the same in both the acute and chronic condition, these changes in dopamine-blocking effects without interference with the therapeutic action suggest either an alteration in sensitivity of some central dopamine mechanisms or a compensatory change in other transmitter systems.

There is evidence that 7-hydroxychlorpromazine is an active (that is, antipsychotic) metabolite and its concentration shows a correlation with clinical improvement. Conversely chlorpromazine sulphoxide is not active, and some non-responders produce relatively large amounts of this metabolite.

In some investigations chlorpromazine plasma levels of 35–350 ng/ml have been associated with clinical improvement and the ratio of CPZ + 70H–CPZ/CPZ–SO>1 in most good responders. Severe toxicity develops with levels above 600 ng/ml.

Actions and side-effects Chlorpromazine is a typical member of the neuroleptic phenothiazines. It possesses moderately powerful sedating, anticholinergic, alpha-adrenoceptor blocking, antiemetic and antipsychotic activities. Parkinsonism, acute dystonic reactions, akathisia, perioral tremor and tardive dyskinesias may all complicate treatment.

As with all neuroleptic agents, spontaneous motor activity is reduced, and this action combined with rigidity and bradykinesia may imitate catatonia. However, true catatonia in schizophrenics is relieved by chlorpromazine.

The effect of chlorpromazine on sleep is unpredictable but the drug usually has sedating properties. Other sedatives given concurrently are potentiated. In delirious states and other disturbances which interfere with sleep, chlorpromazine can restore more normal sleep patterns. EEG patterns are altered in both normal and psychotic individuals; there is a slowing and decrease in variability in frequencies (synchronization) – the proportion of theta (θ) and delta (δ) waves is increased, alpha and fast beta waves are decreased. There may be a net increase in wave amplitude. Alpha wave increases due to sensory stimuli are blocked by chlorpromazine.

This drug is particularly prone to reduce seizure threshold and increase EEG activity often associated with epilepsy (see page 138). Chlorpromazine most frequently precipitates overt fits in epileptic patients and in addicts who are being withdrawn from alcohol or hypnotic drugs.

Failure of ejaculation, usually without impotence, is commonly caused by chlorpromazine (see Chapter 9).

Jaundice is a more common toxic effect of chlorpromazine than of therapy with the newer neuroleptics. This is most likely to develop in weeks 2–4 of treatment, but in only 2–4 per cent of patients. The jaundice is the result of a hypersensitivity reaction and is caused by centralobular cholestasis.

Chlorpromazine treatment is associated with agranulocytosis in a frequency of less than 1 in 10 000 of patients; 5 per cent of patients receiving chlorpromazine suffer urticaria or other rashes (including petechial and maculopapular eruptions). Chlorpromazine is particularly implicated in the production of light sensitivity and subsequent grey-blue skin pigmentation. The drug can similarly cause deposits in the cornea and lens and lead to pigmentary retinopathy.

Uses

- Excited psychotic states: for example, acute schizophrenia, mania and hypomania, delirium.
- Severe anxiety and panic.
- Terminal illness, in particular potentiation of the action of opiates in the alleviation of the distress due to pain.
- Alpha-adrenoceptor blockade; used in the treatment of shock and in hypertensive reactions produced by monoamine oxidase inhibitors.
- Antiemetic in metabolic disease (such as uraemia), terminal illness, opiate and cytotoxic drug therapy, X-irradiation.
- Antihiccough.
- Premedication and part of the medication in neuroleptanalgesia; also used to produce hypothermia in cardiovascular surgery.
- Huntington's chorea – used for its antipsychotic and antichorea properties.

Promazine

This phenothiazine has an aliphatic side-chain and has similar properties and uses to chlorpromazine. It has the reputation of being more sedating than chlorpromazine and is used by some psychiatrists for the treatment of excited episodes which occur in the course of senile dementia.

Thioridazine

Thioridazine is a neuroleptic phenothiazine with a piperidine ring in the side-chain attached to the nitrogen of the phenothiazine nucleus.

Pharmacokinetics Plasma protein binding of thioridazine is 96–99 per cent. During redistribution following administration the alpha phase $t_{1/2}$ is 4–10 hours. This is followed by an elimination phase with a $t_{1/2}\beta$ of 26–36 hours. On fixed dose regimes there is at least a tenfold variation in steady state levels. The elderly, in particular, show elevated plasma levels compared with the young.

Thioridazine is metabolized to a side-chain sulphone and sulphoxide. When these two substances are administered to schizophrenic patients they are less effective than the parent compound and are associated with a higher incidence of side-effects.

As with chlorpromazine it has not been clearly established whether plasma levels of thioridazine are correlated with clinical response in schizophrenia.

Actions and side-effects Thioridazine possesses the usual actions of the neuroleptic phenothiazines. Its piperidine side-chain confers considerable sedating properties and powerful alpha-adrenoceptor and cholinergic muscarinic receptor blockage. The alpha-blocking properties increase the risk of significant hypotension with orthostatic fainting. The elderly in particular are vulnerable to such postural hypotension. Although the anticholinergic effects predispose to constipation and hesitancy of micturition, this action reduces the parkinsonism which occurs due to dopamine receptor blockade, and because of this, parkinsonism is less frequent and less severe than with the other phenothiazine neuroleptics.

Pigmentary retinopathy is particularly prone to develop with thioridazine – but only with high doses such as an excess of 1000 mg daily.

Uses Thioridazine is useful in psychotic states with considerable excitement and agitation. Although effective in excited noctural episodes in the elderly (and less likely to produce extrapyramidal toxicity than the other phenothiazines) thioridazine can predispose to falls (and hence injury) because of severe postural hypotension.

Piperazine phenothiazines

These are powerfully antipsychotic drugs but do not possess the sedative properties of chlorpromazine, promazine and thioridazine. They are particularly prone to produce parkinsonism but trifluoperazine and thiopropazate are used in chorea and some other dyskinesias. They are all very effective antiemetics – prochlorperazine suppresses vestibular function in Ménière's disease; trifluoperazine is used in drug-, radiation- and metabolic-induced nausea and vomiting. Trifluoperazine may be used as an alternative to metoclopramide and domperidone in migraine to suppress nausea and allow the effective administration of analgesics (see Chapter 12).

BUTYROPHENONES

This group of drugs has properties similar to the piperazine phenothiazine neuroleptics described above. They are powerfully antiemetic and are prone to produce extrapyramidal toxicity. They do not usually produce profound sedation.

Antipsychotic butyrophenones

Drug	Dose	Special uses
Haloperidol	0.5–5 mg orally 8–12 hourly Up to 30 mg intramuscularly 6-hourly	Tranquillization in acute psychotic excitement, especially mania; Gilles de la Tourette syndrome; withdrawal from narcotics; premedication
Benperidol	0.25–1.5 mg orally daily	Deviant and antisocial sexual behaviour
Droperidol	2–20 mg daily orally 5–10 mg intramuscularly or intravenously	Premedication and neurolept-analgesia; antiemetic
Trifluoperidol	0.5–2.5 mg daily orally	Tranquillization in acute psychotic excitement, especially mania

Haloperidol

Haloperidol is a butyrophenone which was synthesized by Janssen and first shown to be effective in psychosis in 1959[4]. Its structure resembles pethidine but its actions are similar to trifluoperazine.

Pharmacokinetics The bioavailability of orally administered haloperidol is about 50–70 per cent; the elimination $t_{1/2}$ is 10–19 hours – elimination is slowed during sleep. Unlike the phenothiazines, haloperidol is not an enzyme inducer. On regular dosing there is a linear relationship between daily dose and plasma steady state levels.

Haloperidol appears to be itself antipsychotic and its oxidized products are inactive. In the liver haloperidol is converted to hydrophilic carbonic acids by oxidative dealkylation. These are excreted and conjugated with glycine.

Many patients whose psychotic illness responds to haloperidol have plasma levels of 3–10 ng/ml, but some patients only improve when considerably higher levels have been attained.

Actions and side-effects Haloperidol is less sedating than chlorpromazine but more prone to produce parkinsonism. In one series in which large doses were used, extrapyramidal toxicity developed in about 80 per cent of the patients. It is powerfully antiemetic and results in less postural hypotension than chlorpromazine.

THIOXANTHINES

This group of neuroleptics is said to possess some antidepressant activity, although this has yet to be shown unequivocally. The degree of sedation which they produce is unpredictable, and some patients experience stimulation. The group produces alpha-adrenoceptor blockade, anticholinergic activity and extrapyramidal toxicity to a similar degree as chlorpromazine. The antipsychotic drugs in this group include:

- Chlorprothixene orally 30–400 mg daily (divided doses).
- Flupenthixol orally 0.5–3 mg daily, intramuscularly 20–200 mg every 2–4 weeks.
- Clopenthixol intramuscularly 200–400 mg every 2–4 weeks.
- Thiothixene.

DIPHENYLBUTYLPIPERIDINES

These include:

- Pimozide orally 2–20 mg daily.
- Fluspirilene intramuscularly 2 mg weekly.
- Penfluridol.

Although this group of drugs is powerfully antipsychotic, only little sedation is produced and there is minimal alpha-adrenoceptor blockade and anticholinergic activity.

DIHYDROINDOLES

Antipsychotic drugs with indole structures include:

- Oxypertine orally 80–120 mg (divided doses).
- Molindone.

These drugs are moderately sedating, show little extrapyramidal toxicity and minimal alpha-receptor blockade.

DIBENZODIAZEPINES

- Clothiapine.
- Clozapine.
- Loxapine.
- Metiapine.

Clozapine has little neurological toxicity but may show some bone-marrow toxicity.

As a whole the group is moderately anticholinergic but has minimal extrapyramidal effects.

Sulpiride shares many properties with drugs of this group but is an orthopramide. The dose is 400–800 mg daily.

DEPOT NEUROLEPTICS

Neuroleptics may be injected intramuscularly in depot form (usually as esters) and given at intervals of 1–4 weeks. The main advantage of this technique is that many of the problems of patient compliance are removed. Some of the neuroleptics (such as chlorpromazine) show high first metabolism with much variation in bioavailability. Much more reliable absorption occurs following intramuscular injection of the following:

- Fluphenazine decanoate.
- Fluphenazine enanthate.
- Flupenthixol decanoate.
- Clopenthixol decanoate.
- Fluspirilene.

Case history: depot neuroleptics (1)

After leaving school at the age of seventeen, a boy obtained a job as a clerk in a hospital works department. He did well and enjoyed his work for two years. After this time he became argumentative and sullen, and was asked to leave. He continued to live at home but underwent a change in personaltiy – instead of being friendly and cheerful, he became quiet and distrustful. He slept during the day and went to a weightlifting gym in the evenings. He sometimes went for one- to two-hour runs in the early morning. Several months after leaving work he began to complain to his parents that a 'gang' followed him in a car when he went running; he bought a knife 'to defend himself' but on several occasions threatened his parents. A doctor was consulted and he was admitted to hospital. Schizophrenia was diagnosed and neuroleptic therapy started. Treatment was changed several times – the patient was found to be a poor complier with oral medication. Finally, reasonably acceptable social behaviour was restored on large doses of a depot preparation – fluphenazine decanoate 250 mg intramuscularly every three weeks, although this resulted in considerable emotional flattening. He has not worked since the start of his illness.

Case history: depot neuroleptics (2)

A shy girl of nineteen from an academic family worked well towards her pre-university A-level examinations. During her first paper (English literature) she became unable to continue with the exam and left the examination room. She felt she could no longer think and had lost her energy, but could not further explain her actions. She did not proceed with any more exams and left school. Three years later she managed to find work in the office of a small hotel. She carried out her duties satisfactorily but had no social life at all apart from occasionally attending a students' Christian group.

At this time she began to attend several doctors' surgeries and a hospital outpatient clinic, and also consulted a faith healer. Her complaints were that she suffered from discomfort due to a nail lodged in her spine. She said this was put there by a German paratrooper who sexually assaulted her when she was an infant. Several X-rays of her spine failed to reveal any abnormality. This did not reassure the patient. On direct questioning she sometimes described hearing male voices which were unpleasant and 'bossy'.

She was admitted to hospital and improved rapidly on being given chlorpromazine, although she became apathetic. She was therefore discharged on a more stimulant neuroleptic – intramuscular flupenthixol decanoate 40 mg every 4 weeks. Although she appeared to be well on this regime, she felt that the psychiatrist had made a mistake in his diagnosis, and would only agree to continuation of treatment if he reduced the dose to 10 mg every 4 weeks. On this dose the worry about the nail in the spine, feelings of loss of energy and constant thoughts about the German paratrooper all returned. However, she is now back at work and her problems are not known to her supervisor in the hotel.

EXTRAPYRAMIDAL AND OTHER SIDE-EFFECTS OF NEUROLEPTICS

The common side-effects of the neuroleptics have been documented earlier in this chapter, but particular mention must be made of the extrapyramidal and associated disorders.

All known neuroleptics block central dopamine actions. The neuroleptics available do not select between various dopamine systems in the brain and will block those involved in the psychotic process (the mesolimbic pathway) in addition to those involved with coordination of fine movements (nigrostriatal pathway).

Side-effects resulting from blockade of dopamine receptors in caudate nucleus

- Acute dystonic reactions
- Akathisia
- Extrapyramidal side-effects
- Tardive dyskinesias

Acute dystonic reaction

This occurs in a small number of patients (1–4 per cent) and can occur shortly after administration of the very first dose.

The most typical is the oculogyric crisis which consists of rolling up of the eyes in spasm, twisting of the neck as in torticollis, and protrusion of the tongue. Response to intravenous drug treatment is dramatic: procyclidine (20 mg), orphenadrine (100 mg) or benztropine (20 mg) will usually produce a complete reversal in a matter of minutes. The addition of intravenous diazepam (5–10 mg) will potentiate this treatment. Usually diazepam alone is effective, although it can be hazardous by this route.

Akathisia

The patient experiences subjective feelings of restlessness and anxiety, and is often totally unable to sit still. While the traditional treatment is the administration of anticholinergic medication, its efficacy is now in question, and altering the drug dose or changing medication may be necessary.

Extrapyramidal side-effects

This common side-effect of the neuroleptics, parkinsonism, takes the form of rigidity (cogwheel type), akinesia (minimal movements, with typical mask-like face) and tremor ('pill-rolling', resting type). The response to antiparkinsonian anticholinergic medication (such as benzhexol, benztropine, procyclidine) should alleviate symptoms without stopping the drug. There is no reason to prescribe anticholinergic medication routinely, and it is now believed to sensitize patients to the development of tardive dyskinesia.

Tardive dyskinesia

First described in 1957, this movement disorder is found in 15–35 per cent of patients receiving continuous neuroleptic medication. It takes the form of facial movements, choreo-athetoid trunk and limb movements, and leg movements which might be difficult to distinguish from akathisia. The major problem with this serious side-effect is its delayed onset associated with poor response to any conventional drug treatment.

It is currently held that the condition is due to dopamine receptor hypersensitivity, which could explain the exacerbation of symptoms on stopping the neuroleptic, and some transient easing of symptoms when prescribing an even more potent dopamine blocker, often followed by even more severe tardive dyskinesia. As with all current thinking on receptors in the brain, the theory has its critics and some findings, inconveniently, do not fit. From a purely practical viewpoint, we are no nearer a treatment for this potentially disabling condition. Tardive dyskinesia is particularly serious as there is the social stigma attached to bizarre facial and body movements. Paradoxically, while using neuroleptics to maintain schizophrenics in the community and prevent psychotic breakdown, the treatment itself confers on a percentage of schizophrenics the further burden of yet another social handicap.

NEUROLEPTICS AND BEHAVIOUR

Neuroleptic medication is extremely effective in controlling the florid, active or positive symptoms of schizophrenia, but less useful in dealing with the negative symptoms such as social withdrawal, flattening of affect, lack of motivation and, as in the most severe cases, general personality deterioration. It is in these areas that social treatments play a vital role. Rehabilitation of the chronic schizophrenic patient in conjunction with behavioural treatment for specific disabilities is the mainstay of treatment.

In association with neuroleptics, the treatment of schizophrenics involves physical, behavioural, psychological and social techniques.

NEUROLEPTIC USE IN OTHER CONDITIONS

Neuroleptics have a potent antipsychotic action and are useful in a wide range of psychotic conditions other than schizophrenia.

Neuroleptic medication is used in many cases of acutely disturbed behaviour, but not before a complete history has been obtained.

Acute organic psychoses

Acute organic psychoses may manifest signs and symptoms including hallucinations, delusions, clouding of consciousness, mood disturbances, extreme restlessness and a fluctuating course. There are many causes of such a picture and these include vital organ failure, metabolic and endocrine disturbances, infections, substance abuse and drug withdrawal. The treatment of such disturbances is that of the underlying cause and also, symptomatically, with neuroleptics.

Alcohol withdrawal

Alcohol withdrawal is a common cause of an acute organic state and can present with the typical syndrome of delirium tremens (see Chapter 7). In alcohol withdrawal it is preferable to use chlormethiazole or a benzodiazepine rather than a neuroleptic, because of the propensity to develop grand mal seizures and the high incidence of liver damage.

Paranoid psychoses

Paranoid psychoses apart from schizophrenia may also be treated with neuroleptics (possibly depot injections), often in the long term if the condition is recurrent. As would be expected, considerable skill is needed to retain the confidence of a paranoid patient and ensure compliance with the medication.

Extra care is needed to keep doses to the minimum which are effective. Paranoid patients generally tolerate even the mildest side-effects poorly, and often stop their medication because of this.

Paraphrenia of old age Elderly patients suffering from these discrete paranoid states may require maintenance medication even though they are unreliable drug-takers. While there is a temptation to give depot neuroleptic medications by injection, the elderly are particularly vulnerable to side-effects, which can be increased by intercurrent infection, and because the depot dose is not flexible. Depot neuroleptic medication in the elderly is therefore contraindicated except in exceptional circumstances.

Manic patients

These respond rapidly to neuroleptics (see Chapter 3). In a small proportion of very agitated depressive patients phenothiazines may be indicated, although not in the long term.

PRACTICAL POINTS

- Most schizophrenic patients are diagnosed and established on medication in hospital. The aims of treatment are to return the patient back to home and work as soon as possible, and to relieve distressing symptoms.
- Aggravating factors (such as family problems and examinations) should be reduced as much as possible.
- Drugs are the main physical treatment, and this consists of oral therapy (e.g. chlorpromazine) or depot neuroleptics (e.g. fluphenazine enanthate). The particular advantage of depot neuroleptics is that they remove many patient compliance problems, schizophrenics usually being poor in this respect. But medication should be reviewed regularly, particularly in long-term therapy.
- ECT is used for associated depression or to shorten phases of excitement.
- Chlorpromazine is the main drug used in treating schizophrenia, but thioridazine (and possibly promazine) are favoured in the elderly.
- All neuroleptics block dopamine receptors and share extrapyramidal and associated side-effects to a greater or lesser extent.
- Routine anticholinergic medication is not advised.
- The dose of neuroleptic should be titrated in each patient in order to achieve the desired effect. The dose may be built up if the expected response is not forthcoming.

3
Drug treatment in affective disorders

BACKGROUND

The vast majority of patients who are treated for affective disorders are seen only by their general practitioners, and few ever see a psychiatrist. Many of these patients have non-specific problems which do not constitute classical depressive illness, but present with various depressive symptoms, anxiety, or general irritability.

A problem in the treatment and assessment of affective disorder is the use of the word 'depression'. The term is used medically to describe a specific syndrome or illness, while in a non-technical sense it embraces anything from feelings of loss, unhappiness, anxiety, inability to cope, to severe melancholia. This is a major cause of confusion, and until the doctor and patient have agreed a common language, a reasonable and accurate assessment of the situation cannot be made. In order to avoid this area of misunderstanding, it is important that the patient can explain himself not in terms of phrases such as, 'I am depressed', but by describing exactly how he feels. This may in fact reveal that the patient is not suffering from depression at all.

This semantic difficulty with the exact meaning of the word 'depression' has led to increasing use by the medical profession of the terms 'depressive illness' or 'affective disorder' to describe that group of patients where feelings of sadness and their accompanying symptoms go beyond what might be considered normal and enter the realms of the morbid state.

A diagnosis of affective disorder or depressive illness is not solely dependent on lowered mood, which is, after all, only one symptom in a complex cluster making up the range of disorders under consideration.

LIFE EVENTS AND DEPRESSION

The relationship between unpleasant life events and depression is well documented and has been widely investigated in the population at large. The best-known study relating problems identified as depressive with life stresses took place in South London in a largely working-class inner city area[5]. Not only was there a class difference in the prevalence of depressive symptoms, but within the groups where these symptoms predominated, they appeared to be most severe in women with young children who were isolated and lacked intimate social and family contacts. Having an unsympathetic spouse further complicated matters. It is easy to predict that many women who fulfil these criteria will ultimately present at the general practitioner's surgery complaining of a variety of symptoms, but most commonly, a cluster identified by the patient as depressive. These women rarely respond to antidepressant drugs, and social intervention is more applicable in these cases. Whether this takes the form of social work and services, psychiatric district services by nurses or aides, or by general practitioners themselves, depends on local resources. Local support groups to assist in dealing with just such problems have sprung up over recent years (see the Useful Addresses section at the end of the book).

MANAGEMENT OF DEPRESSION

Once the first hurdle of deciding whether the patient is suffering from true affective disorder is cleared, the next step is to decide upon the appropriate course of treatment. To achieve this, the classification of depressive illness has to be brought under scrutiny. A diagnosis is of little practical use if it does not give the physician some idea of treatment and outcome.

In our present state of knowledge the identification and classification of depressed patients and prediction of response to treatment relies mainly on clinical judgement. The main aim of research into diagnosis and classification is towards an ideal situation in which clusters of symptoms enable clinicians to predict response to treatment and thus influence the choice of treatment.

At the most basic level depression is commonly divided into 'neurotic' and 'endogenous'. Before discussing these in more detail, it is worth noting that the majority of patients presenting with an affective disorder do not slot neatly into one category of the other, and share features of both, making treatment decisions and absolute diagnosis considerably more complicated.

Depressive neurosis

The neurotic type of depressive illness has often been called 'reactive'. This leads to confusion, as endogenous depression, too, may well follow significant life events.

Characteristic features The characteristic features of the depressive neurosis are sleep disturbances, usually associated with worry, typically manifesting as difficulty in getting off to sleep. Frequently there is an appetite disturbance without significant weight loss, although there may be a tendency to excessive food intake. In addition there are significant symptoms of anxiety with increased reactivity of mood in which the patient's affect is excessively vulnerable to external environmental influences.

Suicidal ideas are common, and the risk of overdose is high. Patients who talk about suicide may be labelled as 'manipulative', but these patients at times do succeed in killing themselves and should be taken seriously (see page 36).

Underlying factors in depressive neuroses always have to be considered, whether they are situational, such as relationship problems or social crises, or due to personality difficulties associated with inadequacies in coping mechanisms or emotional immaturity. There may well be a long history of hysterical-type behaviour, obsessional or anxiety symptoms and a diagnosis of chronic depressive neurosis. Depressive neuroses respond poorly to antidepressant medication.

Treatment The major treatment thrust in this group is social intervention, associated with psychological support, best offered by the general practitioner with the assistance of a nurse therapist or social worker in those group practices geared for this.

Depressive neurosis varies greatly in severity, and in cases where there is a poor response to the psychological and social intervention described, or where there are some features which overlap with a diagnosis of endogenous depression, antidepressant medication may be indicated, although the response is usually not good. These patients are particularly vulnerable to the hazards of long-term prescription of benzodiazepine drugs.

Endogenous depression

True endogenous depressive illness with the classical presenting symptoms of early morning wakening, diurnal variation of mood (low in the morning and improving through the day) and poor appetite associated with loss of weight is not as common as depressive neurosis. There may be a family history of depression or a past history of discrete episodes of an affective disorder with response to either antidepressants or electroconvulsive therapy (ECT). A combination of such features suggests that the patients could show a good response to antidepressant drugs.

Unfortunately, the clinical presentation is seldom clearcut in this way, and many patients also have symptoms of a depressive neurosis.

Laboratory tests It has been suggested that the group of patients whose symptoms are strikingly 'biological' (that is, endogenous, non-neurotic) show differences in results of some laboratory tests from those in other patients[6]. One of these is the dexamethasone suppression test (DST). The response to administration of oral dexamethasone is usually a total suppression of cortisol secretion. In endogenous depression is it proposed that there is associated overactivity of the pituitary–adrenal axis whereby the normal response to dexamethasone is abolished, and cortisol levels remain elevated. This unusual response to dexamethasone occurs in 60 per cent of endogenous depressive patients. In some patients the DST may provide a diagnostic aid and also monitor the response to treatment.

Psychotic features There are often psychotic features in severe depressive illness. These may take the form of depressive hallucinations or nihilistic and persecutory delusions associated with poor insight. Severe agitation may be superimposed on the depressive features of the illness. Typically, these patients are admitted to hospital early and often receive ECT with concomitant antidepressant therapy. There might be an indication in the most agitated or psychotic patients for the addition of a neuroleptic drug (see Chapter 2).

Treatment The treatment of choice for endogenous depressive illness is physical (mainly antidepressant drugs), with concomitant and later supportive psychotherapy to assist with adjustment. A problem in endogenous depression, particularly when there is some retardation, is the high risk of suicide when the patient starts responding to treatment, as there may be an improvement in motivation and energy without the attendant disappearance of suicidal thoughts. The treating physician always has to bear this in mind, particularly when prescribing potentially toxic medication.

Case history: endogenous depression

Soon after Christmas, a fifty-three-year-old schoolteacher, Mr P.W., started feeling lethargic and generally lacking in energy. His concentration was poor, and when he returned to school after the Christmas holiday he felt less able to function. He felt that he was somehow letting people down, particularly his wife and children. Food became less appetizing to him, tasting flat and sometimes unpleasant, and he lost interest in his appearance. His wife noticed that he was losing weight and developing a 'haggard look'. He would sit for long periods looking into space, or alternatively, would pace up and down, wringing his hands. His sleep was becoming progressively more disturbed with restlessness and early waking. He felt unable to cry, although he felt sad, and he tended to feel a little brighter in the evenings. His marriage was a supportive one. There was no evidence of any past history of mental illness.

He first visited his general practitioner in the middle of January, and presented his complaint as one of sleep disturbance. It was clear at this time that his mood was depressed, and on questioning, all the symptoms of a classical endogenous depressive illness were elicited. He was commenced on imipramine, 50 mg at night, increasing to 150 mg daily, and was asked to return to the surgery after two weeks.

He did not respond to this treatment. He continued to deteriorate and became more agitated at times, with longer periods of being withdrawn and uncommunicative. He was admitted into a psychiatric unit with a diagnosis of endogenous depression with stupor. He resisted taking food and liquids and was physically retarded.

The treatment of choice in this case was ECT, which was instituted as a life-saving measure, with the agreement of both his wife and an independent consultant. The ECT was given three times weekly to a total of eight, and his recovery was rapid and complete. As soon as he was able to take tablets he was established on an adequate dose of a tricyclic antidepressant, in this case amitriptyline (see page 46), which was monitored by measuring plasma concentrations. This was done to ensure that an adequate concentration of antidepressant was present in the blood without unnecessary and time-wasting dosage adjustments.

He was discharged from hospital four weeks after receiving the first treatment. His medication was discontinued after twelve months. In view of the severity of the problem and its fairly rapid onset, and increasing dose of a tricyclic antidepressant was appropriate (for example 50 mg amitriptyline for one week increasing to 150 mg over the next two weeks), particularly if he was able to stay off work. A more sedative drug such as amitriptyline is most useful if one of the symptoms of the depressive illness is sleep disturbance. The medication could be given in one fixed dose at night.

A male patient of this age and with this presentation is always a significant suicide risk and it is often desirable at the very earliest stage to refer him to a specialist clinic with a view to possible rapid admission to hospital. Often patients refuse this, and the family should then be vigilant, in particular keeping control of the medication. The patient himself should be expected to pay regular visits to the practice. Of course if suicidal intent is communicated in the context of a depressive illness of this sort, compulsory admission to hospital may need to be considered. Plasma concentration estimation is still a luxury in many centres, but if available it is particularly useful in monitoring tablet compliance and in helping to avoid drug toxicity.

Depression in the elderly

The elderly consume more psychotropic drugs than any other age group, and may react quite differently to drugs generally, when compared with younger people.

Special problems Depression in the elderly presents special problems, not least in its diagnosis. It must be differentiated from dementia (see Chapter 5) and various physical disabilities such as myxoedema and Parkinson's disease. Adverse drug reactions, particularly to tricyclic antidepressants (which can cause a toxic confusional state, hallucinations or agitation), are common over the age of sixty, and potentiation of glaucoma or retention of urine associated with prostatism may prove special problems. In addition, because of the cardiotoxicity of these drugs, they are contraindicated in ischaemic heart disease and in patients with cardiac arrhythmias.

It would appear that the newer antidepressants which have been shown to be effective, such as nomifensine, trazodone and mianserin (see page 48), would be most suitable in the elderly, being low in troublesome anticholinergic effects and lacking in obvious cardiotoxicity.

For the elderly as a group significant depressive illness may be more appropriately treated with ECT in the first instance in view of the problems experienced with antidepressant medication.

THE CHOICE OF AN ANTIDEPRESSANT

There are many antidepressants presently on the market (see pages 40–1) and the choice is a perplexing one.

All the tricyclic antidepressants share certain features: they all have anticholinergic side-effects to a greater or lesser extent; they all potentiate noradrenaline peripherally; and they may be cardiotoxic in large doses. No one tricyclic carries an obviously smaller risk of cardiotoxicity than another. (Doxepin, which has been claimed to be the least cardiotoxic tricyclic, shares similar properties with the others when administered in equivalent doses.) The newer non-tricyclic antidepressants such as mianserin, nomifensine and trazodone, are much less toxic and are less dangerous in overdose.

Toxic and side-effects of antidepressants

In practice the choice of antidepressant is often dictated more for differences in toxicity of the drugs than for the types of depression to be treated. For example many tricyclics and mianserin are sedative, and while they are never used primarily for sleep disturbance, the skilful prescription of these drugs at night will reduce the need for hypnotics in depressed patients. Most tricyclics may be prescribed in a single dose at night which probably reduces some of the side-effects during waking hours. Toxic effects tend to disappear as the drug becomes effective and the patient experiences a lifting of the depressed mood.

Nomifensine is useful in patients susceptible to grand mal seizures. It is not sedating and can be given as a single daytime dose.

In patients with prostatic hypertrophy or glaucoma the relative lack of anticholinergic properties of mianserin, nomifensine and trazodone favours the use of these antidepressants.

Monoamine oxidase inhibitors (MAOIs)

The monoamine oxidase inhibitors were the first antidepressants to be introduced. In recent years, with the introduction of safer antidepressants, the MAOIs have become less popular and are now reserved for use in phobic anxiety states where there is a suspected underlying depressive illness, and as part of the treatment of refractory depressive illness in combination with tricyclics. In combined antidepressant therapy (MAOIs and tricyclics) – a potentially dangerous therapy – only specific combinations should be used, such as phenelzine and trimipramine.

The MAOIs are no longer first-line antidepressants and their infrequent use is confined, in the main, to psychiatric units (see page 50).

PLASMA LEVELS OF ANTIDEPRESSANT DRUGS

Plasma level assay for drugs is now widely available in many hospitals.

For plasma level monitoring of drugs the criteria which are particularly applicable to antidepressants can be summarized:

- Where there is a proven relationship between drug concentration and clinical efficacy
- Where there is a wide variation of plasma levels between individuals
- Where the drug has a low therapeutic index, that is, where the difference between therapeutic levels and toxic levels is small
- To determine drug compliance

Because there is no agreement whether there is a clear relationship between plasma levels of antidepressants and therapeutic response, there is at present no reason to include drug levels in the usual drug treatment of depressed patients, apart from the routine measurement of lithium levels in all patients on this drug (see pages 57–61).

There is a relationship, however, between high plasma levels and side-effects, resulting in poor compliance and, on rare occasions, serious physical effects.

With these drugs there is a poor relationship between the dose prescribed and the level measured. In some academic centres blood levels of tricyclic and other polycyclic antidepressants are carried out during treatment in order to assess compliance, interpret toxic effects and identify whether patients who fail to respond are rapid metabolizers of the drug.

Blood level estimations are not available for the MAOIs.

MAINTENANCE MEDICATION

Once a patient has shown a good response to antidepressant medication, continuation with the drug is indicated, and acts to protect the depressive from further breakdown. The suggested time scale is six months to one year on the drug, though studies investigating this are few and difficult to conduct[7].

ECT does not, as a rule, replace antidepressant medication, and only in exceptional circumstances where drugs are contraindicated, will antidepressant medication not be started as an adjunct to ECT to ensure a better long-term response to treatment.

In bipolar depressive illness lithium is the maintenance drug of choice (see later pages). Tricyclics and other antidepressants may precipitate manic attacks in these patients.

SUICIDE AND DEPRESSION

The overall incidence of successful suicide has decreased slightly in recent years, although there has been a great increase in attempted suicide. The fall in suicide rate is most likely due to the increased vigilance of medical practitioners resulting in earlier and successful treatment of depressive illness. In addition, there has been a distinct change in prescribing patterns, with toxic medication being less freely available. The group of patients that successfully commits suicide is strongly associated with depressive illness, and is therefore eminently treatable. Patients who have attempted suicide unsuccessfully belong to a much more heterogeneous group, including some with depressive illness, many with personality disorders, and many seemingly well-adjusted people whose suicide attempts were made in response to stress.

There is, of course, overlap between the groups. Some people do kill themselves when not clinically depressed, and, fortunately, many calculated suicide acts associated with depression do not succeed.

Suicide profile

The person who attempts suicide is very often a young female with some histrionic, immature or inadequate personality traits, social crises in the recent past, a history of previous overdose or other acts of self-harm and with evidence of impulsive behaviour. While it seems that patients in this group are not suffering from classical depressive illness, experienced clinicians in this field identify in many individuals shortlived bouts of severe lowered mood, pessimism and anxiety.

As clinical studies are conducted it is also evident that the response to antidepressant medication in this group is extremely poor[6]. We, as practitioners, have a responsibility not to prescribe toxic medication to patients who have threatened or attempted suicide.

At-risk patients

The at-risk depressed patients who kill themselves have most often visited their general practitioners in the months prior to the act. The alarm bells should sound when older men in their 50s and 60s who have started complaining of depressive symptoms, where there may be physical illness, alcoholism or impending or recent retirement or divorce. The tragedy of missing treatable depression in these cases is immense. Of course, depressive illness and associated suicide is not the exclusive domain of this group, and vigilance is clearly indicated in all patients with depressive symptoms no matter the age or sex.

Treatment

Treatment of depressive illness where there is a strong possibility of a suicidal act is best carried out in hospital. In some instances, when urgent change in mood is required, ECT is considered. As mentioned already, partially treated patients with some retardation may well become an increasing suicidal risk as the depression lifts.

BEREAVEMENT AND DEPRESSION

Grief is a normal phenomenon and as such does not require medication. A typical grief reaction may pass through a characteristic sequence. Initially there is an act of denial followed by shock and restlessness. This is replaced by apathy and a feeling of numbness which may progress to final acceptance.

A common association with grief reactions is a massive increase in consultations with the general practitioner, particularly by young widows.

Psychological and somatic complaints at these visits can range from illusions and pseudohallucinations to insomnia, headaches and generalized bodily aches and pains.

Atypical grief reactions

These occur mainly in women and usually last longer than one year. There is an increase both in suicidal ideas and attempts at suicide. There is often strong denial of the problem and its atypical nature can cause some diagnostic problems.

Treatment

Treatment in atypical grief reactions is mainly psychological, working with the patient through the normal stages of grief.

Antidepressant therapy is sometimes indicated, particularly if there are more typical symptoms of a depressive illness or if the symptoms are particularly severe or resistant to psychological management.

UNIPOLAR AND BIPOLAR MOOD CHANGES

Dividing depressive psychoses into unipolar and bipolar has become increasingly popular in recent years. Unipolar includes recurrent endogenous depressive illness, whereas bipolar describes that group of manic-depressive psychoses manifesting both depressive and manic bouts. There is often evidence of a strong family history in this group, with the clear suggestion of a genetic component. A diagnosis of unipolar depression may have to be changed to bipolar if hypomanic mood swings develop. This highlights yet again the difficulties encountered when attempting to offer an unequivocal diagnostic classification.

When treated in a depressive phase, the bipolar group responds to antidepressant medication or ECT, and in a manic bout to neuroleptics and lithium. Maintenance of these patients is with lithium treatment (see later), and once commenced may be continued for many years.

Mania

Mania is characterized by an increased wish to communicate (called 'pressure of speech' in psychiatric jargon) and flight of ideas associated with physical hyperactivity. In its mildest form it may be barely detectable, while in its severest, it is uncontrollable and is associated with paranoid delusions.

Management Patients may suffer from bouts of recurrent mania, or manifest mood swings of the bipolar type. In either case the management of acute attacks of mania is with neuroleptics in most cases, and the long-term prophylactic treatment of choice is lithium. The control of hypomanic or manic episodes with neuroleptics, such as chlorpromazine, is often dramatic. Lithium is itself effective as a treatment for mania in addition to its mood-stabilizing qualities in prophylaxis and maintenance. The decision to commence lithium therapy as maintenance treatment in recurrent mania is made with the same care as with bipolar or recurrent depression. The principles of lithium treatment are discussed in detail at the end of this chapter.

DRUG ACTION IN DEPRESSION

Drugs which ameliorate depression potentiate the availability and effectiveness of amine transmitters in brain synapses (see Figure 3) – although the various types of antidepressants do this in different ways. For example, the tricyclic antidepressants, trazodone and maprotiline inhibit neuronal reuptake of amines from the synaptic cleft

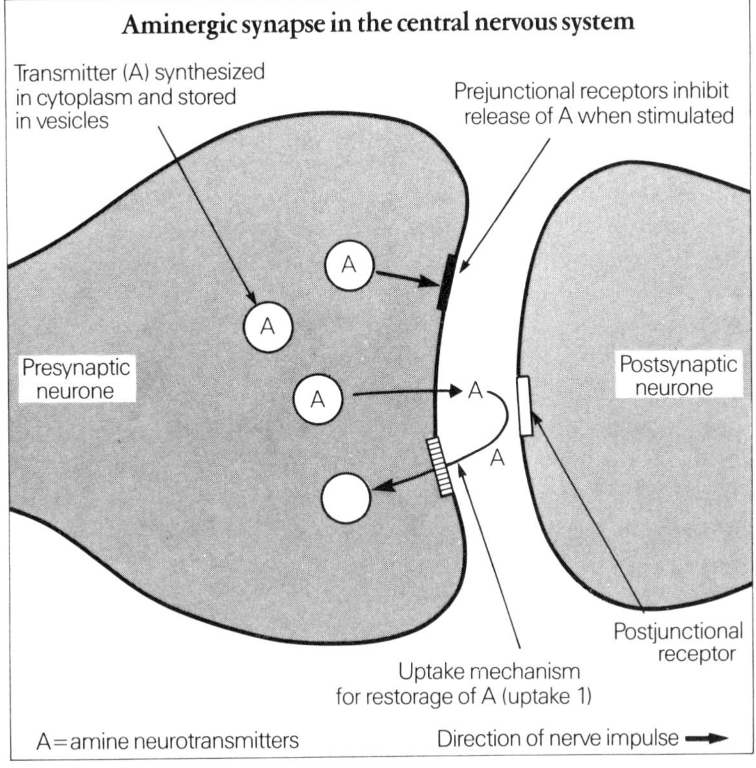

Figure 3 According to the amine theory of mood, depression results from reduced stimulation of postjunctional receptors.

(see Figures 4 and 5); the MAOIs raise the total amount of brain amines (see Figure 7); and mianserin increases amine transmitter release from nerve endings (see Figure 6).

Antidepressant drugs: classification

- Tricyclics (iminodibenzyls, dibenzocycloheptenes, anxiolytic tricyclics)
- Tetracyclics
- Miscellaneous structures, e.g. nomifensine, trazodone
- Monoamine oxidase inhibitors (MAOIs)
- L-tryptophan
- Hormones and vitamins, e.g. L-triiodothyronine, thyroid-stimulating hormone (TSH), oestrogens, pyridoxal phosphate
- Thioxanthines
- Lithium

TRICYCLIC ANTIDEPRESSANTS

All these antidepressants block the neuronal uptake of noradrenaline, 5-hydroxytryptamine (5-HT) or dopamine. The tricyclic antidepressants all possess an amine side-chain – the tertiary amines mainly block noradrenaline uptake.

The tricyclic antidepressants are variably sedating and potentiate the actions of alcohol. In addition they share several other properties:

- Anticholinergic: dry mouth, constipation, hesitancy in micturition, blurring of near vision, aggravation of glaucoma, delayed orgasm, impotence
- Sympathomimetic: cardiac arrhythmias in overdose
- Epileptogenic: large doses can provoke fits and pharmacological doses may aggravate pre-existing epilepsy

Tricyclic antidepressants: 1. Iminodibenzyls

Drug	Dose (taken at night)	Structure and activity	Active metabolite	$t_{½}$ (h)	Special features
Imipramine	50–300 mg	Tertiary amine; equally powerful inhibition of noradrenaline and 5-HT uptake	Desmethylimipramine ($t_{½}$ = 12–24 hours)	4–18	Usually sedating but can produce insomnia; powerful anticholinergic
Trimipramine	50–150 mg	Tertiary amine; predominantly inhibits 5-HT uptake, metabolite blocks noradrenaline uptake	Desmethyltrimipramine		Very sedating; moderately anticholinergic
Clomipramine	50–150 mg	Tertiary amine; inhibition of 5-HT uptake	Desmethylclomipramine, potent noradrenaline uptake inhibitor	Dose-dependent kinetics	Sedating
Desipramine	50–300 mg	Desmethylimipramine — a secondary amine; inhibition of noradrenaline uptake		12–24	Characteristic of secondary amines: little sedation, less anticholinergic activity than seen with tertiary amines

Tricyclic antidepressants: 2. Dibenzocycloheptenes

Drug	Dose	Structure and activity	Active metabolite	$t_{1/2}$ (h)	Special features
Amitriptyline	50–150 mg	Tertiary amine; powerful inhibition of 5-HT uptake, some effect on noradrenaline uptake	Nortriptyline ($t_{1/2}$ = 18–96 hours)	8–24	Powerful sedative; powerfully anticholinergic
Butriptyline	25–50 mg three times a day	Tertiary amine; weak inhibitor of noradrenaline and 5-HT uptake	Present	70–140	
Nortriptyline	50–150 mg at night	Desmethyl-amitriptyline: secondary amine; powerful inhibitor of noradrenaline uptake, some effect on 5-HT uptake		18–96	Mildly sedating, weakly anticholinergic
Protriptyline	15–60 mg at night	Secondary amine		50–200	Usually mildly sedating, may be stimulant; moderately anticholinergic

Tricyclic antidepressants: 3. Anxiolytics

Drug	Dose (taken at night)	Active metabolite	$t_{1/2}$ (h)	Special features
Doxepin	50–150 mg	Desmethyldoxepin ($t_{1/2}$ = 30–72 hours)	8–24	Less powerful antidepressants than amitriptyline and imipramine; has anxiolytic activity
Dothiepin	75–200 mg		48–60	As doxepin above
Maprotiline	50–150 mg		24–60	Has a basic tricyclic structure to which is added a methylene bridge to form a ring perpendicular to the rest of the molecule. Its main bio-chemical action is inhibition of noradrenaline reuptake, with a lesser effect on 5-HT uptake. It has anticholinergic and cardiotoxic effects as do the rest of the tricyclics, and may cause grand mal seizures

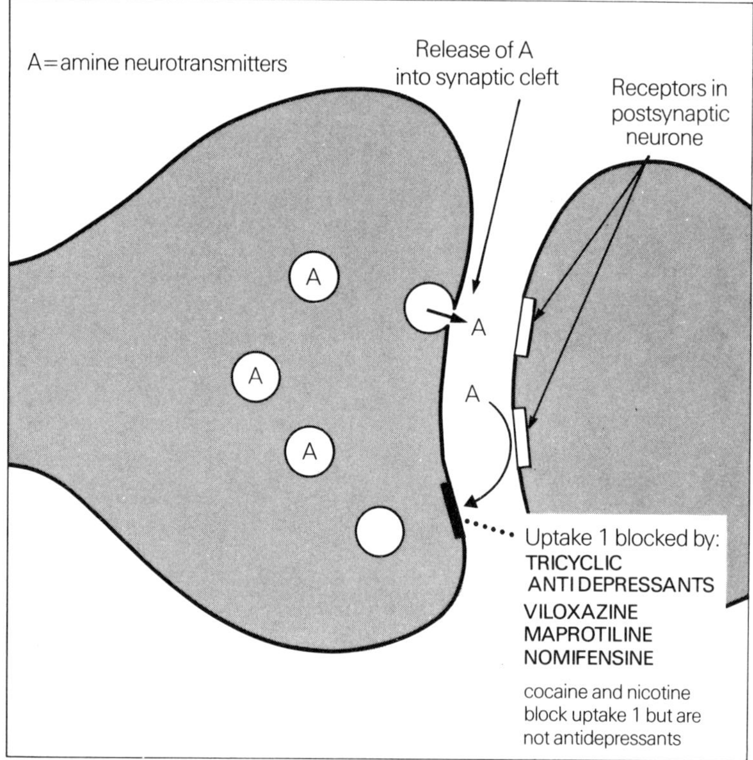

Figure 4 Uptake 1 is the main mechanism by which amine transmitters are removed from the synapse. Many antidepressants raise synaptic concentrations of amines by producing a block in uptake 1.

- Long $t_{1/2}$, high plasma protein binding, large volume of distribution (for example, imipramine V_d = 28–61 l/kg), some metabolites are active
- Optimal therapeutic response is usually delayed for two to three weeks after starting treatment

Toxic effects

Apart from the highly dangerous consequences of overdose, serious side-effects are uncommon.

Common side-effects

- Anticholinergic effects
- Cardiovascular: postural hypotension, palpitations
- Overdose: supraventricular tachycardia, ventricular tachycardia, A–V block, bundle branch block, prolonged PR, QRS, QT intervals, T wave flattening, ST depression
- Central nervous system (CNS): sedation, heavy sleep and difficulty in waking, disturbed sleep, myoclonic jerks, tremor, choreiform movements, headache; the appetite may increase.

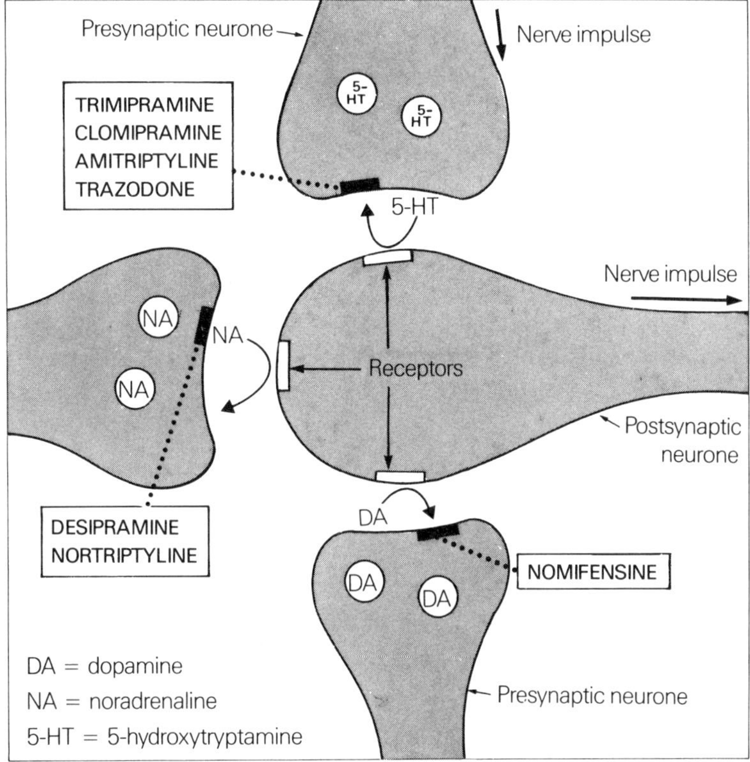

Figure 5 Many antidepressants act by blocking uptake 1 of various amine transmitters. This diagram shows some of these drugs which have a selective action on individual amines.

Uncommon but serious toxic effects

- Anticholinergic: paralytic ileus, acute retention of urine
- Cardiovascular: sudden death, presumably due to ventricular fibrillation
- CNS: fits, acute confusional psychosis, hypomania
- Alimentary: cholestatic jaundice
- Haematological: thrombocytopaenia
- Allergic: angio-oedema, light sensitivity

Drug interactions

A most important interaction is that the sedation produced by the tricyclics is potentiated by other central depressants, which include alcohol, neuroleptics and hypnotics.

The usual doses of MAOIs if taken with usual doses of tricyclics produce hypertension, hyperpyrexia and excitement and can also lead to coma, cerebral haemorrhage and death. Techniques have been developed in some specialist centres to administer these drugs concurrently (in small doses) for refractory depression. Such procedures are potentially dangerous and should not be used by the non-specialist.

Central stimulants, such as the amphetamines, can precipitate excitement, hypertension and cardiac arrhythmias in patients taking tricyclics.

The tricyclic antidepressants abolish the hypotensive actions of clonidine, debrisoquine and bethanidine. Lithium tremor may be increased by these drugs.

Contraindications to tricyclic antidepressants

- Recent myocardial infarction; cardiac arrhythmias; cardiomyopathy
- Pregnancy (if at all possible to withhold treatment)
- Atony of gut or bladder, bladder neck obstruction
- Epilepsy
- Liver or renal failure
- Glaucoma

Imipramine

Iminodibenzyl was synthesized in the late nineteenth century. The pharmacological properties of iminodibenzyl derivatives were first investigated in 1948. One derivative – imipramine – was at that time found to have sedative properties. Imipramine differs structurally from promazine, the neuroleptic phenothiazine, only by replacement of the sulphur in the central ring of the nucleus with an ethylene linkage. In tests on psychotic patients in the United States in 1958, R. Kuhn found that it was ineffective in excited and agitated states but discovered by chance that it was effective in some depressed patients. Subsequent clinical trials by Kuhn revealed that imipramine was effective in endogenous depression, but could sometimes aggravate reactive neurotic depressive illness[8].

Imipramine is the parent drug to all the other tricyclic antidepressants described subsequently in this chapter, and for this reason is covered in greatest detail.

Pharmacokinetics Following oral administration imipramine is completely absorbed but undergoes a considerable but variable first-pass metabolism. The range of bioavailability is 29–55 per cent. This variation is independent of the variability in $t_{1/2}\beta$. The reduced bioavailability of imipramine following oral administration is completely explained by increased formation of desipramine (an active metabolite) and other inactive metabolites. Imipramine absorption is complete from the intestine in eighty minutes and no metabolite formation occurs in the intestinal wall. Desipramine is detected in the peripheral blood ten minutes after administration. This indicates that demethylation occurs in the liver – desipramine is the desmethyl metabolite of imipramine. There is evidence of an enterohepatic circulation for imipramine and desipramine.

Absorption has been compared between oral and intramuscular administration. Earlier and higher peak levels are recorded after intramuscular injection compared with the oral route. Also, following intramuscular injection less desipramine appears in the plasma.

Following absorption, imipramine is highly protein bound (87.7 ± 7.4 per cent) but, again, there is considerable interindividual variation. The range of free drug is 5.5–23 per cent and it is presumably this form which enters the cerebrospinal fluid. Because of this it has been postulated that free antidepressant drug concentrations may be better correlated with clinical efficacy than are the total drug concentrations, more usually estimated.

The tricyclic antidepressants are present in very low concentrations in the plasma and their apparent volumes of distribution are large, presumably due to extensive tissue binding. However there is much individual variation in $V_{d\beta}$. For imipramine the $V_{d\beta}$ varies between 28–61 l/kg. This varies inversely with the fraction of unbound drug, so that the ratio $V_{d\beta}$/(free drug in plasma) is a constant and is approximately equal to 3.

The half life ($t_{½\beta}$) for imipramine varies widely. After a single oral dose it is found to be 4.0–17.6 hours but after multiple doses lies between 9.2 and 20.2 hours. One explanation of these observations could be non-linear kinetic behaviour. Even bigger variation is seen for the main active metabolite, desmethyl imipramine (3.5–16.5 hours).

The variability in pharmacokinetic properties of these drugs results in great variations in steady state plasma levels on multiple dosing. There is a tenfold variation in plasma steady state imipramine concentrations in patients on a fixed daily dose of 3.5 mg/kg. The range of plasma levels is 95–1000 ng/ml (mean 210 ng/ml). The contributions to such individual variation in blood levels include interindividual constitutional differences in hepatic metabolism (including first-pass metabolism), variation in apparent volumes of distribution and protein binding in the plasma, and the state of induction of the drug-metabolizing enzymes. It has been shown that other drugs which are oxidized by the liver exhibit similar variation – for instance, there is a close positive correlation between the $t_{½}$ of phenylbutazone and the steady state values of imipramine and desmethylimipramine in a group of subjects on a fixed daily dose of imipramine. Much of the variation in steady state levels of these compounds can be explained by differences in the genetically determined ability of the body to oxidize drugs, although contributions are also made by enzyme induction (particularly by hypnotics, alcohol and nicotine) and by differences in volume of distribution.

Because imipramine, like other tricyclic antidepressants, has a long half life, once-daily administration is probably adequate and sustained-release preparations are unnecessary. On repeated dosing it is expected to reach steady state plasma levels in about a week; thus the more prolonged delay in therapeutic response which usually occurs is not due to attainment of particular blood levels of imipramine but to alterations in the brain produced by the drug.

Actions Imipramine is a typical member of the tricyclic antidepressant group of drugs. Prominent anticholinergic effects are produced. The therapeutic index is small (about 3–4), and in overdose produces dangerous cardiac tachyarrhythmias, fits and paralytic ileus.

In normal volunteers imipramine is usually sedating – but in some depressed patients a stimulant effect may be experienced and insomnia can result.

Uses Apart from its application in depressive illness, imipramine may be helpful in the management of enuresis. Its mode of action in this condition is not understood, but the depth of sleep may be reduced or there could be a local action on the bladder. Imipramine has surface-acting local anaesthetic properties and in the urine could partially anaesthetize the bladder and depress the detrusor reflex. Small doses of imipramine should be used for this purpose as children are particularly vulnerable to the cardiotoxic and epileptogenic actions of this type of drug.

Clomipramine

Like imipramine this is a tertiary amine tricyclic drug with predominantly sedative properties. It appears to act by inhibition of uptake 1 of 5-HT and not of noradrenaline.

Pharmacokinetics Following oral administration peak levels of clomipramine are attained at 2–4 hours, and of the active metabolite demethylchlorimipramine at 4–8 hours. Excretion is slow – the drug can be detected in the plasma for at least 48 hours and in the urine for 14 days. The elimination does not follow first-order kinetics, but appears to be dose-dependent. Intersubject variation of plasma levels on a given dose may be up to fourteenfold. Over 90 per cent of the drug is bound to protein in the plasma; no correlation has been established between plasma level and clinical response.

Desipramine

Desipramine is desmethylimipramine, a secondary amine administered for the treatment of depression. Its blockade of uptake 1 mainly involves noradrenaline. 90 per cent is bound to plasma protein. The elimination half-life varies between 3.5 and 16.5 hours. As with many of the secondary amine tricyclics it is less sedating than amitriptyline and possesses less anticholinergic activity.

Amitriptyline

Amitriptyline is one of the most sedating and is probably the most powerfully anticholinergic member of the series. Nevertheless it is the most widely used and most thoroughly tested of the tricyclics. In depressive illness of the endogenous type 70–75 per cent of attacks are terminated within 3–4 weeks of starting treatment.

The mean elimination half-life is 14 hours (range 9.0–30.5 hours) and in the plasma 96 per cent is protein bound.

Uses Apart from depression, amitriptyline is being investigated in the management of depression in alcoholism, terminal illness and dementia, in phobic-anxiety syndromes and in some cases of obsessive-compulsive neurosis.

Nortriptyline

This is a secondary amine with only mildly sedating and anticholinergic effects.

Pharmacokinetics Following oral administration nortriptyline has a bioavailability of 46–59 per cent. All of the loss is accounted for by the formation of metabolites, the main ones being 10-hydroxy nortriptyline and its conjugates (glucuronide and sulphate); 95 per cent is protein bound in the plasma. The free drug is present in equal concentrations in plasma and cerebrospinal fluid. The volume of distribution is large and the usual range is 29–36 l/kg body weight. The elimination half-life varies greatly between individuals, the range being 18–55 hours. Such variation produces a broad range of plasma levels on repeated dosing; on a repeated dose of 50 mg the steady state plasma level showed fivefold variation (mean 140 ng/ml; SD = 50 ng/ml). This variation is inherited and is under polygenic control. Thus children tend to have mid-parental values and there is much better concordance for identical twins than for non-identical twins.

From a single oral dose it is possible to predict the steady state level and therefore find the daily dose that is needed to give a particular blood level. This can be done in a similar fashion to the method used for lithium (see page 58), since the steady state nortriptyline level can be predicted from a single level taken 24 or 48 hours after a single 100 mg test dose and the dosage is then adjusted accordingly to produce the appropriate plasma concentration. For an individual the optimal dose remains constant over long periods. This is because $t_{½\beta}$ and V_d, which mainly depend on genetic factors that are separately inherited, tend to remain constant.

There is much support for the existence of a curvilinear relationship between therapeutic response and plasma nortriptyline concentration, in that the best outcome is associated with plasma concentrations between 50 and 200 ng/ml. Poor responses are usual at levels lower than 50 ng/ml or in excess of 200 ng/ml. There is nothing remarkable about such behaviour, as it is common knowledge that too little drug produces no response and too much is toxic.

Maprotiline

This is a tetracyclic antidepressant with similar actions to the tricyclics. In fact, a molecular model of this drug shows a typical tricyclic structure plus a methylene bridge over the central ring. It is thus not a true tetracyclic structure, as is mianserin.

Pharmacokinetics On a fixed daily dose of 75 mg, considerable individual variation in plasma steady-state levels has been observed (30–230 ng/ml). Fits occur with higher doses and this toxic effect is usually associated with plasma levels above 200 ng/ml. Clinical response has been noted at levels between 18 and 155 ng/ml but further studies are required to delineate the response curve for this drug. Maprotiline is highly protein bound but there is broad variability as to its extent in different individuals. The substance is well absorbed following oral administration and the first-pass hepatic metabolism is apparently unimportant. There is a long half-life (27–58 hours) and thus

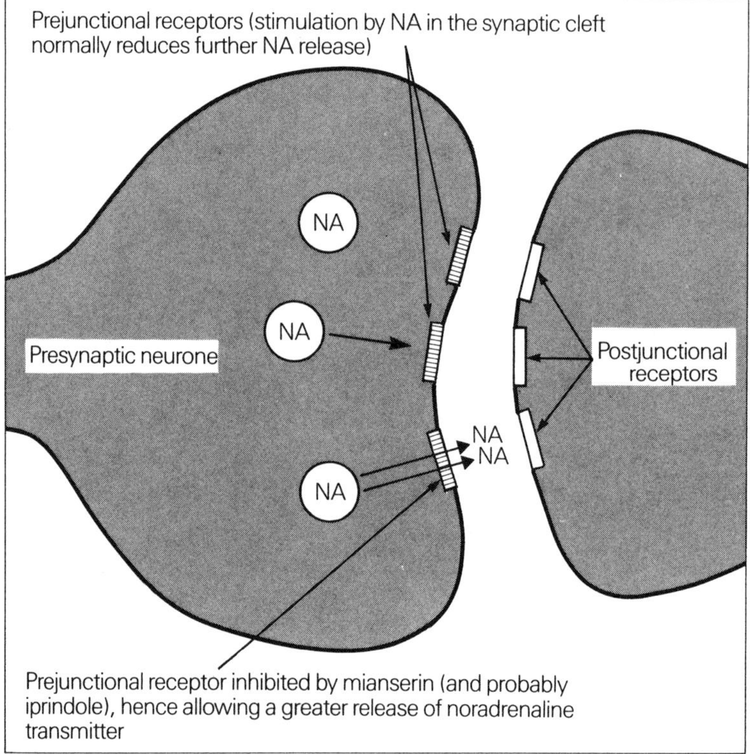

Figure 6 Mode of action of mianserin in enhancing the release of noradrenaline into the synaptic cleft. It is possible that prolonged treatment with tricyclics produces its antidepressant action because of a delayed reduction in the sensitivity of prejunctional receptors, thus enhancing the release of amines into the synaptic cleft.

steady state plasma levels are not attained until the second week of treatment.

In overdose, like the tricyclics, maprotiline produces sympathomimetic effects on the heart, powerful anticholinergic actions, and fits.

TETRACYCLIC ANTIDEPRESSANTS

Mianserin

This is the only true tetracyclic antidepressant in general use.

In addition to presynaptic adrenergic blockade (alpha-autoreceptor blockade) with potentiation of noradrenaline release there is some postsynaptic 5-HT receptor blockade.

Pharmacokinetics Mianserin is rapidly absorbed after oral administration with peak concentrations being achieved at 2–3 hours. The half-life of redistribution is 1.4 hours and the mean elimination half-life is 10 hours (range 7.7–19.2 hours) so that steady state after repeated doses is achieved in 3–4 days. Most of the dose is metabolized in the liver by aromatic hydroxylation, *N*-oxidation and *N*-demethylation. Only 4–7 per cent is present in the urine in unchanged form. Hepatic first-pass metabolism reduces the oral bioavailability to 30 per cent. One investigation showed that patients with plasma mianserin levels above 70 ng/ml and below 15 ng/ml have a poorer clinical response than those within this range. Single dose experimental studies have correlated sedation and slowing of the EEG rhythm with the height of mianserin blood levels.

Toxicity In overdose, mianserin is considerably safer than the tricyclics as it has no sympathomimetic action on the heart and is not anticholinergic. There are sedative properties, but unless another central depressant is taken concurrently, death does not usually result from overdose. In therapeutic doses postural hypotension is common. Fits can be precipitated. Reversible neutropenia has been described in a few cases.

Administration A single evening dose of 30–80 mg.

MISCELLANEOUS STRUCTURES

Viloxazine

This bicyclic antidepressant has similar properties to the tricyclic drugs. It is anticholinergic and can produce cardiac arrhythmias or, in large doses, fits. In addition, toxic effects which often limit the dose are nausea or headache. Similarly its mode of action is inhibition of amine uptake – having an equally powerful effect on 5-HT and noradrenaline reuptake processes.

Pharmacokinetics Viloxazine has a short elimination half-life (2–5 hours) because of almost complete metabolism. The main metabolites are a hydroxyl derivative of both rings, and of the aromatic ring only which appears in the urine as glucuronide conjugates. During the first 24 hours after administration 98 per cent is excreted in the urine and 2 per cent is recovered in the faeces. Peak levels in the plasma bear a linear relationship to the oral dose and are roughly 0.8 μg/ml plasma per mg/kg body weight viloxazine. Peak levels occur at 1–4 hours. The drug is not highly protein bound. The usual total daily dose is 150–300 mg.

Nomifensine

The structure of this drug is vaguely tricyclic but it is a phenylisoquinoline and does not have a phenothiazine-like molecule. However, its mode of action causes a powerful blockade of noradrenaline and dopamine uptake, and there is also a weak inhibition of 5-HT uptake.

Pharmacokinetics Nomifensine has a short half-life (1.5–2 hours) due to extensive and rapid metabolism. This may be prolonged up to 46 hours in renal failure. After oral administration peak levels occur at about 1½ hours. However, it is mainly the metabolites which are detected in the plasma in a ratio of about 40:1. The free aromatic ring forms monohydroxy derivatives at the 3 and 4 positions, 3-methoxy-4-hydroxy and 3-hydroxy-4-methoxy derivatives and several conjugates of these. It is not known if any of these are active.

Uses Nomifensine is not sedating. It is usually stimulating and much less anticholinergic and sympathomimetic than the classical tricyclics. In overdose there is little cardiotoxicity. The usual dose range is 75–200 mg daily. The recommended dose is one 100-mg tablet in the morning. It has little effect on convulsant threshold – there may even be a reduction in proneness to fits. Because of this, nomifensine may be useful in depression in epileptic patients.

Iprindole

This has a classical tricyclic structure but with an indole nucleus and cyclo-octane ring. The action of this drug is unique in that it blocks the reuptake of noradrenaline in the brain, but does not have such action peripherally.

In addition to antidepressant activity iprindole is anxiolytic; it is a mild sedative and has weak anticholinergic properties. The dose is 30–60 mg, 8-hourly.

Trazodone

This is a triazolepyridine. In low concentrations it is a 5-HT antagonist, but in higher concentrations it has 5-HT receptor stimulatory activity because of blockade of 5-HT uptake.

The drug is completely absorbed from the gut and is almost completely metabolized to inactive compounds. The plasma half-life is 3–5 hours. Trazodone is sedating and anxiolytic but has very weak anticholinergic properties and little cardiotoxic potential in overdose.

MONOAMINE OXIDASE INHIBITORS (MAOIs)

The monoamine oxidase inhibitors raise the total brain content of amines, including noradrenaline, 5-HT and dopamine. This happens because cerebral mitochondrial monoamine oxidase is inhibited. As this is one of the routes of amine destruction within the neurone, there is a progressive rise in concentration of these transmitters. Unfortunately amine stores in the peripheral sympathetic nervous system are also augmented, and also some exogenous amines are not adequately metabolized in the body. These two additional effects can give rise to dangerous reactions and greatly limit the use of this type of drug.

The rise in brain noradrenaline, like other centrally acting α-agonists, produces a reflex hypotension. The build-up in brain amine stores is produced by a temporary imbalance in breakdown and synthetic processes. It then takes up to two to six weeks to establish the new increased level of amine stores. In parallel with this, the clinical improvement may be delayed by two to six weeks.

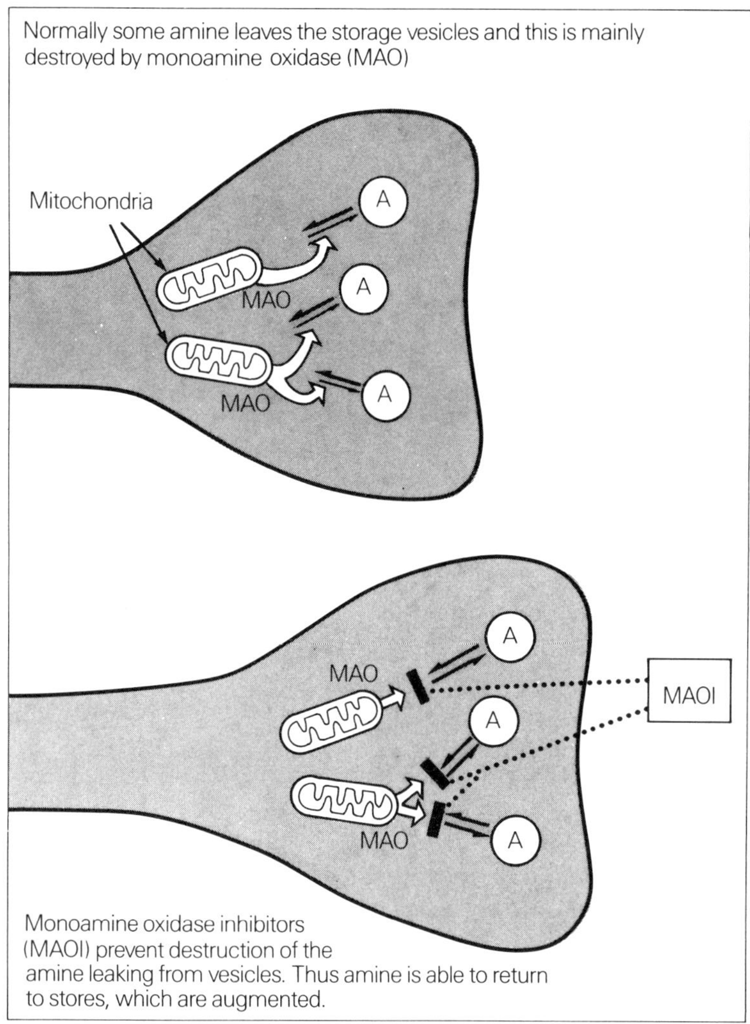

Figure 7 Monoamine oxidase inhibitors act as antidepressants by increasing amine transmitter stores in presynaptic nerves.

Iproniazid

Isoniazid and iproniazid (isopropyl isoniazid) were shown to be very effective antituberculous drugs in 1951[8]. An advantage of these over streptomycin is that they penetrate the blood–brain barrier and can therefore be used in the treatment of tuberculous meningitis. Within a few months of its introduction several physicians had noticed that iproniazid (but not isoniazid) had mood-elevating properties in tuberculous patients. In 1952 J. Delay and P. Deniker published the results of a trial carried

Major MAOIs in use

Drug	Single tablet (mg)	Daily Dose (mg)
Hydrazines		
Iproniazid (effective but use limited by hepatoxicity and production of peripheral neuropathy)	50	100–250
Phenelzine (most commonly used MAOI in depression; can cause drowsiness)	15	45–120
Isocarboxazid	10	39–90
Non-hydrazine		
Tranylcypromine (stimulatory – can cause insomnia and amphetamine-like effects)	10	20–60

out in France showing the effectiveness of iproniazid in depressed (non-tuberculous) patients. Shortly afterwards this work was confirmed in several centres and it was also shown that iproniazid (but not isoniazid) was an inhibitor of monoamine oxidase[9].

This series of discoveries was important from several points of view:

1. Iproniazid was the first drug which had a significant action in any of the major psychoses.
2. The fact that a simple chemical agent influenced a functional psychosis supported the possibility that such mental illness could have a biochemical basis.
3. If the significant difference between iproniazid or isoniazid was the monoamine oxidase blocking property of iproniazid, then a hypothesis could be constructed implicating cerebral monoamines as being involved in mental illness and, more specifically, a depletion of amines being the underlying lesion in depressive psychosis.

Since that time the amine theory has expanded to include other mental illnesses and there has been some elaboration as to the amines involved. However, the field is a difficult one and biochemical data is sparse and as yet inconclusive.

Pharmacokinetics Biopsy and blood samples show that on continuous treatment with iproniazid maximum inhibition of monoamine oxidase is not attained for five to ten days. The molecule is cleaved to give active products and these bind irreversibly to monoamine oxidase and to some other enzymes concerned with oxidative metabolism of foreign compounds. On cessation of therapy the effect of the inhibitor persists for two to three weeks (that is, until new enzyme molecules are synthesized). Like other hydrazides the drug is metabolized to an inactive acetyl derivative – the extent to which this is carried out is inherited in a simple Mendelian manner. About one-half of the population of western Europe and North America are slow acetylators and require lower doses of the drug. Middle Eastern populations contain a much higher proportion of rapid acetylators.

Uses Although iproniazid is one of the more effective monoamine oxidase inhibitors in the treatment of depression, it is mainly used when other drug treatment has failed. This is because of its ability to cause acute hepatic necrosis and peripheral neuropathy. Toxicity apart, iproniazid is probably less effective than the tricyclic antidepressants.

Phenelzine

This is a hydrazide derivative. It is inactivated by acetylation and slow acetylators suffer an increased risk of acute hepatic necrosis when the drug is given in usual doses.

Although phenelzine cannot readily be measured in the blood, this is probably unimportant because its action on tissue enzymes is its essential manifestation. When phenelzine has attained 75–80 per cent inhibition of blood platelet monoamine oxidase, antidepressant activity may appear (albeit after a delay of one to three weeks).

Uses Apart from use in endogenous depression, phenelzine may be beneficial in reactive (neurotic) depression – even when tricyclic antidepressants have failed. It may also be useful in the treatment of phobic anxiety and in dysphoric neurotic states.

Isocarboxazid

There is little evidence that this drug is an effective antidepressant.

Tranylcypromine

This non-hydrazine MAOI is one of the most active antidepressants in this group. Nevertheless, it has not been shown to be more active than the tricyclic drugs.

Uses As with phenelzine and iproniazid, tranylcypromine is only used when, in a patient with depressive illness, adequate doses of tricyclic antidepressants over a period of five to six weeks have failed and ECT has been refused.

The drug is also used in phobias, intractable anxiety and dysphoria. MAOIs are all-powerful inhibitors of paradoxical or rapid eye movement (REM) sleep, and may prove to be useful in the treatment of narcolepsy.

Toxic effects of MAOIs

Food and drug interactions are the most serious dangers with the MAOIs; other toxic effects are less frequently encountered than with the tricyclic antidepressants.

- **Nervous system**
  Neurological: Headache, aggravation of migraine, drowsiness, tremor,

weakness, paraesthesiae, peripheral neuropathy, muscle spasm, ataxia, fits

Psychiatric: Nightmares, insomnia, nervousness, confusion, hallucinations, hypomania, aggravation of schizophrenia

Autonomic: Dry mouth, constipation, hesitancy of micturition, retention of urine, impaired accommodation of near vision, impotence, delay or failure of orgasm, postural hypotension, sweating

- **Alimentary system**
  Hepatocellular damage, anorexia, nausea, vomiting

- **Metabolic disturbances**
  Increased antidiuretic hormone (ADH) secretion, oedema, weight gain, hypoglycaemia

- **Bone marrow**
  Leucopenia

Food interactions

Foods which contain indirectly acting sympathomimetic amines can produce hypertension, headache, cerebral haemorrhage, hyperpyrexia, fits, coma and death. The most dangerous is matured cheese (which contains tyramine). Tyramine is also present in some wines (Chianti, for example) and beers (especially Bass and Worthington in Britain). Broad-bean pods contain dopamine; meat and yeast extracts contain mixtures of amines including histamine.

Other foods which have produced hypertensive reactions in patients taking or recently withdrawn from MAOIs include:

- Bananas (especially the skin)
- Game
- Pickled herrings
- Green figs
- Fish roe

Drug interactions

1. Indirectly acting sympathomimetics can produce fatal hypertensive reactions. Even the small amounts of ephedrine or phenylethylamine which are absorbed into the circulation from decongestant nose drops have caused a hypertensive crisis. When these agents or amphetamine are taken by mouth, serious toxicity is the rule in patients taking MAOIs.
2. Directly acting sympathomimetics such as adrenaline, noradrenaline or phenylephrine do not usually produce serious hypertensive reactions.
3. Levodopa is a potent cause of hypertension in patients on MAOIs.
4. Although tricyclic antidepressants are used in combination with MAOIs by experts in treating refractory depression, this can be a dangerous and even lethal combination.

5. The MAOIs block a range of oxidizing enzymes, including those which inactivate narcotics (especially pethidine), barbiturates, phenytoin, oral hypoglycaemic agents and chloral. The effects of these drugs are prolonged and enhanced. Although adverse effects can be experienced with alcoholic beverages, this is probably due to the amines formed during fermentation.
6. The inactivation of some hypotensive agents and muscle relaxants may also be inhibited and their action is increased.
7. Acute confusional states may develop with anticholinergic drugs (such as benztropine), tetrabenazine and methyldopa.

Case history: tranylcypromine interaction

A twenty-nine-year-old man had been on tranylcypromine 10 mg twice daily for two months when he developed severe pleural pain. He was seen at home by his general practitioner, who administered 100 mg pethidine intramuscularly, having made a provisional diagnosis of a non-tension pneumothorax. While his doctor was explaining the need for an X-ray at the hospital the patient became restless, agitated and incoherent finally lapsing into unconsciousness some ten minutes after the injection. He was transferred to hospital by ambulance where he was found to be flushed (temperature 38°C) and sweaty with a blood pressure of 100/60 mmHg and a sinus tachycardia of 160/min. Cheyne-Stokes respiration was noted and the pupils were dilated and unresponsive to light. No deep tendon reflexes could be elicited and the plantar responses were extensor. Conservative treatment was undertaken after a lumbar puncture was found to be normal. The patient slowly regained consciousness and was discharged well twenty-four hours later.

Commentary Concurrent use of pethidine and MAOIs results in this potentially fatal reaction in certain patients. The mechanism of this sensitivity is not known but there is evidence that the reaction is due to increased levels of 5-HT in the brain. It has been treated successfully with prednisolone or chlorpromazine; and urinary acidification, which enhances MAOI excretion, shortens its duration.

A similar effect has been reported with morphine but this is much rarer and it has been found that some patients on MAOIs who have reacted adversely to pethidine have received morphine without mishap. Rarely dextromethorphan (an antitussive opiate in several cough mixtures) has also produced collapse in patients on MAOIs but methadone has not been reported to produce such effects despite concurrent use.

Pethidine is thus contraindicated in patients on MAOIs unless careful testing for sensitivity, using low initial doses, is undertaken and this is rarely feasible. The interaction of newer analgesics such as nefopam and meptazinol with MAOIs is not yet known.

Overdose of MAOIs

The signs of overdose appear within hours of taking an overdose of MAOIs. The patient may become hypotensive, collapse and enter a state of shock, or conversely may develop an acute hypertensive reaction, possibly with fits due to a hypertensive encephalopathy. The earliest symptoms frequently include anxiety, agitation and hallucinations. In these patients there may be pyrexia and hyperreflexia. Fits can also accompany hyperpyrexia.

Management is difficult. Vital functions must be maintained – in particular, care of the airway, respiration, blood pressure and temperature. Hepatic necrosis may be delayed to up to one week after overdose.

L-TRYPTOPHAN

This has not been shown to be unequivocally antidepressive on its own, but appears to potentiate the effectiveness of MAOIs and of tricyclic antidepressants (particularly those with 5-HT activity, such as clomipramine).

The drug is given in divided doses of 5–9 g daily and is mildly sedating. Otherwise L-tryptophan has low toxicity. Following oral administration L-tryptophan is well absorbed. In normal individuals peak plasma concentrations occur at 1 hour. After a dose of 32 mg/kg body weight, the 1-hour peaks have a mean value of 80 μg/ml (having subtracted the normal tryptophan plasma concentrations which are usually 10–15 μg/ml). Depressed patients have a lower and later peak: 55 μg/ml at 2 hours. In both groups the free tryptophan $t_{1/2}\beta$ was 2.7 hours.

HORMONES AND VITAMINS

L-triiodothyronine, thyroxine and thyrotropin

These have all produced equivocal results in depression but possibly increase the effectiveness of tricyclic antidepressants, although only for specialist use.

Oestrogens

These have been used in intractable depression in women. As their efficacy for this is still unproven, their use is discouraged.

Pyridoxal phosphate (vitamin B_6)

This is used in depression in women taking the contraceptive pill. Its effectiveness has not been convincingly demonstrated.

THIOXANTHINES

These agents have both neuroleptic and antidepressant properties (see page 24). Most neuroleptics are held to have some antidepressant qualities, and this is not surprising considering, for example, the tricyclic structure of the phenothiazines. Thioxanthines, and specifically flupenthixol, are antidepressant in low doses, but a case for use of this drug in primary depressive illness has not yet been satisfactorily made.

LITHIUM

The element lithium (usually administered as the carbonate) is remarkable. Its use has been established as a prophylactic in affective disorders, particularly in preventing abnormal swings of mood (cyclothymia), but also in recurrent unipolar illness (depression or mania). Acute mania also responds to lithium. Lithium is being investigated in the treatment of a number of other disorders including cluster headache, chronic alcoholism and hyperactivity in children.

Pharmacokinetics

Lithium is usually administered as the carbonate, and is well absorbed following oral administration. Capsules and tablets are equally well absorbed, but slow-release preparations show variable absorption in the upper part of the small intestine and can produce diarrhoea and abdominal discomfort due to large amounts of lithium passing to the large intestine. Lithium passes readily into intracellular water and is distributed evenly throughout the total body water. Protein binding is neglible and the ion can be readily measured in the saliva. In the young and in early adult life the elimination half-life is 8–20 hours, but this may lengthen two- to threefold at night. Much higher values (over 30 hours) have been measured in old age. Because of this, elderly patients usually require lower doses of lithium.

Lithium freely enters the renal glomerular fluid by filtration; of this 70–80 per cent is reabsorbed via the proximal tubule. This occurs by a mechanism shared with sodium, so that competition may become significant: when large amounts of sodium are passing down the tubule, lithium reabsorption by the nephron is decreased, while lithium concentrations rise in the plasma when sodium is depleted.

Toxicity As described overleaf the therapeutic index of lithium is low and the plasma lithium concentration has to be near-toxic before a clinical response is produced. Below 0.8 mEq/l produce no therapeutic benefit, and above 1.5 m/q/l toxicity is experienced. (However, dose-independent toxicity such as nausea, diabetes insipidus and goitre can appear within these limits of plasma concentration.) Because of great interindividual variation in the ability to eliminate lithium, the dose a patient may need to attain therapeutic plasma concentrations can be between 1200 and 3600 mg per day. During routine blood level monitoring, samples must be taken exactly twelve hours after the previous dose (on a twice-daily dosage regime). Samples taken early give a spuriously high result.

Plasma level monitoring A further complicating factor which underlines the need for plasma level monitoring is that not only is there individual variation in the magnitude of the peak with a fixed dose of lithium, but also the shape of the plasma concentration/time curve and the time taken to reach peak blood levels both vary considerably. The usual time range for lithium carbonate tablets and capsules to peak is 1–1½ hours and for sustained-release lithium (Priadel) is 5–7 hours. Acceleration of gastric emptying with metoclopramide results in earlier lithium peaks. Delay of gastric emptying with atropine-like drugs can delay the peak for up to 12 hours.

Dosage There are several methods for predicting lithium dosage in individuals by carrying out a preliminary single dose of lithium and measuring serial blood levels afterwards. Some of these are complex and require computing facilities. However, the safest method may be careful dosage increments with repeated 12-hour plasma lithium estimations until the steady state maintenance dose has been found. A single daily dose is usually unacceptable because, although in some patients it may provide adequate plasma levels, peak levels will be high and expose the kidneys to toxic concentrations of lithium, albeit for short periods.

Administration

Lithium carbonate is given orally once or twice daily. One scheme is to start with one tablet daily (each tablet = 300 mg = 8 mmol) and then adjust the dose each week according to plasma levels. The optimum levels for prophylaxis of recurrent affective disorders are 0.4–0.8 mmol/l. For the treatment of mania, levels of 0.8–1.4 mmol/l are considered optimal. The levels are measured 12 hours after the previous dose.

Toxic effects

1. **Adverse effects related to plasma levels** Within the therapeutic range (0.6 – 1.0 mmol/l) a tremor may develop. Above this (1.5–3 mmol/l) the tremor becomes more severe and there may also be diarrhoea, ataxia, weakness and thirst. Above 3 mmol/l these phenomena increase and confusion, spasticity, fits, dehydration and coma may result. Death results from levels of 5 mmol/l or above.
2. **Adverse effects not blood-level dependent** Goitre (with or without hypothyroidism or hyperthyroidism) and renal effects (chronic renal damage and nephrogenic diabetes insipidus). Other dose-dependent toxic effects are cardiac arrhythmias, demineralization of bone and weight gain.
3. **Drug interactions** Diuretics increase lithium blood levels; extrapyramidal toxicity of neuroleptics is increased; metoclopramide accelerates lithium absorption; and atropine-like drugs may delay absorption.
4. **Fetal abnormalities** Lithium may possibly increase the incidence of cardiovascular malformations in the fetus if taken early in pregnancy.

Case history: the dangers of lithium/diuretic interaction

The wife of an architect had five admissions to hospital over five years for a manic-depressive disorder before being started on lithium treatment at the age of fifty-two. For seven years she remained well and was reviewed at six-monthly intervals by her psychiatrist at the local hospital. She was taking sustained-release lithium carbonate (Priadel) 400 mg three times a day and this produced standard 12-hour serum lithium concentrations which varied between 0.7 and 1.1 mmol/l. She was brought to casualty by her husband because over the past 2 weeks she had become apathetic, forgetful and had refused her food complaining of continuous nausea. On examination she had a tremor, was hyperreflexic, and a serum lithium level was reported as 2.7 mmol/l. She was clearly suffering from lithium toxicity and her symptoms resolved when lithium was discontinued. Renal function was found to be normal but upon further enquiry it was found that she had been prescribed bendrofluazide 10 mg daily by a locum general practitioner whom she had consulted for mild ankle oedema.

Commentary Diuretics such as the thiazides decrease sodium reabsorption in the proximal renal tubules thus allowing greater lithium reabsorption to occur at this site. The use of such diuretics in patients on lithium can result in a reduced urine output, paradoxical fluid retention and a rise in serum lithium concentrations. This raised lithium concentration is potentially lethal since the drug has a very low therapeutic index. When diuretic treatment is given to manic-depressive patients on lithium it is important initially to monitor the serum lithium concentration daily (which may require hospital admission), careful supervision being necessary during the first month of therapy.

Principles of lithium treatment

It is reasonable to assume that all patients who might need lithium treatment will have been referred to a specialist clinic, or will have been commenced on the treatment following an acute admission where the diagnosis of bipolar depressive illness is in no doubt.

The decision to stop lithium therapy is a difficult one, and most patients remain on treatment for many years. Thus starting such treatment is a serious step which should only be taken after detailed consideration.

Long-term side-effects The long-term ill-effects of lithium have been highlighted over the past few years[11] and full physical investigations must be carried out before and during treatment, including six-monthly thyroid and renal function tests. Should the patient become hypothyroid, replacement thyroxine can be instituted alongside lithium, particularly where the cessation of lithium results in explosive breakdowns.

If renal function deteriorates then lithium treatment is stopped altogether. Fortunately, overt renal problems are relatively uncommon. Depot neuroleptic medication could be a useful therapy in patients who develop evidence of renal damage.

The low therapeutic ratio of lithium (the plasma level considered therapeutic is very close to toxic levels) means that a close watch must be kept on plasma levels at all times. For this purpose, many hospitals have lithium clinics to monitor their patients. Where these facilities are not available the general practitioner plays an invaluable part in maintaining vigilance.

Some clinicians find that if two or more bouts of depression occur within one year in an elderly person, lithium treatment should be tried. Older patients need a lower dose of lithium to maintain a satisfactory plasma level.

Practical points for lithium therapy

- Treatment is commenced only within the hospital setting, either with inpatients or outpatients
- Maintenance of dose is by repeated plasma level checks, either by lithium clinics or general practitioners
- There are regular (6 monthly) thyroid and renal function tests
- Vigilance is needed when patients complain of toxicity, particularly if these are dose-related effects
- Elderly patients require lower doses

Case history: Successful management of hypomania with lithium therapy

Mr D. P., a forty-six-year-old accountant, was first admitted to hospital at the age of forty. He had been visited at home by his general practitioner at the request of his wife and was found to be exuberant with some irritability, restlessness, emotional lability and rapidity of movement. His speech was so fast as to be almost incoherent and his thoughts were speeded up. He had grandiose ideas about both his capabilities and state of health, and he was lacking in insight.

A diagnosis of hypomania was made and he was admitted to his local hospital. He was started on repeated doses of chlorpromazine 150 mg titrated according to response and settled fairly rapidly. He was discharged after a few days on haloperidol (less sedating) but he developed significant akathisia and the drug was stopped because of this. He was re-established on chlorpromazine, which was found to have less troublesome side-effects in his case, maintained on it for four months, after which it was discontinued. There was no past history of depression, no previous hypomanic episode and no physical cause detected, such as drugs or endocrine disorders.

One year later the problem recurred, with no obvious precipitants. The patient was established on lithium with a diagnosis of recurrent mania. He was maintained on lithium by his general practitioner and had monthly blood lithium estimations and six-monthly renal and thyroid functions tests.

The only bout of mania requiring admission to hospital followed cessation of regular lithium while on holiday. A serious deterioration in his mood and behaviour was narrowly averted at that time, and his lithium concentration was monitored thereafter with extra vigilance. His prognosis is good while he remains on his medication.

PRACTICAL POINTS FOR TREATMENT OF AFFECTIVE DISORDERS

Depression

- Treatment is on an outpatient basis for the majority, with hospital therapy for the suicidal, old, uncared-for, and for severe depression.
- A supportive environment is essential for all patients – in many, sympathy for the patient's suffering may obviate the need for drugs.
- Cognitive therapy can provide long-term help by teaching the patient to curtail his ideas of inadequacy and inferiority.
- When physical therapy is required, supportive psychotherapy should be continued. The main physical treatment is drug therapy. The tricyclics should be tried for at least six weeks, and given in low doses in the elderly. Prostatic hypertrophy or glaucoma are indications to use mianserin, trazodone or nomifensine. Nomifensine is indicated if the patient is epileptic.
- ECT is used particularly if there is a suicide risk.
- MAOIs are used in patients who have not responded to other drugs and for some patients with depressive neurosis.
- Certain foods and beverages (particularly those which contain tyramine) can produce fatal hypertensive reactions in patients taking or recently withdrawn from MAOIs.

Mania

- Admission to hospital is required.
- Drugs are used as early as possible – the neuroleptic phenothiazines are effective, but haloperidol is also widely used.
- Long-term lithium treatment reduces the chance of relapse.

4
Anxiolytic drugs

BACKGROUND

Anxiety is fear which is irrational or out of proportion to the stimulus. It is subjectively unpleasant and generally has physical as well as psychological components. The most common somatic symptoms are dry mouth, nausea, palpitations and tachycardia, shortness of breath, tremor, headache, sweating, paraesthesiae and frequency of micturition. Psychological symptoms range from non-specific worry and irritability to feelings of dread and full-scale panic, in which the main feature is an overwhelming desire to remove oneself from the anxiety-provoking situation as rapidly as possible, associated with feelings of loss of control.

Anxiety, the symptom, is universal. Anxiety states are common and treatable by a variety of means. The major method is not drugs, as is the case in many patients with depression (see Chapter 3).

It is a cause for concern that benzodiazepines are so widely prescribed for such a broad spectrum of problems. There is little evidence that this trend is showing any decline. As with hypnotics, it seems increasingly clear that patients are taught to rely on anxiolytic drugs to alleviate social and interpersonal stresses. This use of anxiety-relieving drugs is counterproductive in such situations.

ANXIETY STATES

Due to the universal nature of anxiety and its prevalence in many psychiatric and medical conditions, the identification and appraisal of morbid anxiety can be difficult.

In acute and chronic anxiety neuroses the symptoms of anxiety are free-floating in nature (in other words, fear not obviously related to any stimulus) whereas in phobic anxiety fear is associated with specific objects or situations.

In some situations a small amount of anxiety can improve performance, but severe anxiety dramatically impairs activity. Such a degree of anxiety transcends that of being an aid to performance and can become intolerable.

In phobic anxiety the symptoms can be directly related to fear of particular objects, as in the specific phobias (animals or insects, for example), but much more commonly there is anxiety about particular situations as in agoraphobia (literally translated as 'fear of the marketplace') or social phobias.

Agoraphobia

Agoraphobia is the most common presentation of phobic anxiety. It is more common in women, typically housewives, who are confined to the home, with significant symptoms associated with venturing out, particularly to busy supermarkets, crowded streets or onto buses. Patients often develop elaborate avoidance mechanisms and in the most serious cases will not leave the home at all. Confrontation with the feared object or situation can precipitate a panic attack, which results in a frightening and usually embarrassing public display. Patients may describe episodes of rapid escape from supermarkets when they have left behind a trail of scattered tins and bemused checkout staff.

Flooding therapy Agoraphobia is treatable with behavioural techniques, although it has a poorer prognosis than object-specific phobias. The most effective method is flooding. In this the patient is progressively but rapidly exposed, in real life, to the situation that provokes his anxiety. The co-operative patient will sometimes deal with the problem alone, but often a therapist is needed. Most agoraphobics improve with behavioural therapy, and there is usually little need for anxiolytic medication.

Specific phobias

More specific phobias are most often treated by systematic desensitization. The feared object is presented, both in imagination and then in real life, in a graduated way, with associated relaxation therapy, both physical and psychological. Sufferers are often very highly motivated, low motivation usually being associated with a poor response to treatment. Most recent studies support the claim that the most successful treatment of phobic anxiety is behavioural therapy.

Chronic anxiety neurosis

This condition is persistent and has few situational or object-specific symptoms. It is often precipitated by relatively minor stresses.

One of the difficulties with the particularly intractable neuroses is that they are associated with personality problems, and this may complicate treatment.

The treatment of anxiety neurosis with free-floating anxiety is usually more difficult than the treatment of phobic anxiety, and may be divided into anxiety management, social skills and assertiveness training, and drug therapy.

Anxiety management The patient develops a regime for dealing with the physical and psychological manifestations of anxiety. The mechanisms for this involve muscular relaxation techniques associated with mental images appropriate to relaxation. Yoga or meditation have similar effects and offer an alternative to hospital-based services.

Social skills and assertiveness training Some patients with anxiety neurosis have significant difficulties in social situations – particularly in being assertive and in gaining self-confidence. Therapy directed towards the development of social skills and assertiveness may be carried out individually, but is usually better handled in group situations with other patients suffering similar problems.

Drug therapy Benzodiazepines (see page 67) are effective anxiolytic agents and useful in the short-term treatment of anxiety neurosis. However, they are widely overprescribed and patients who are given such therapy may find themselves, months or years later, dependent on their medication. As with the hypnotics, it is advisable to ally with the patient, and prevent dependence from developing. This dependence is mainly psychological, but there is clear evidence that with long-term therapy and high doses physical withdrawal signs may also occur. The most serious of these are a toxic confusional state and convulsions. The long-term physical effects of therapy with benzodiazepines are under investigation, and patients who have previously shown a tendency to drug or alcohol abuse should be treated with particular caution. It may be valuable in this group to prescribe small doses of a neuroleptic drug, although their side-effects (see page 26) rule out long-term use except in exceptional circumstances. Apart from the risk of dependence, continuous and regular benzodiazepine administration produces tolerance within a short time, and thereafter little real benefit will be obtained from the medication. Where drug treatment might be necessary in chronic anxiety, intermittent benzodiazepine administration should be encouraged, but the drug should only be used to avert or treat exacerbations of anxiety.

Where physical symptoms such as tremor or palpitations predominate, beta-blockers may be effective, and a small dose of propranolol (40 mg twice a day) or oxprenolol (160 mg daily), both in slow-release form, may be given.

Anxiety states in the elderly

In older patients, before a first-time diagnosis of chronic anxiety neurosis can be made, organic conditions and primary depressive disorders must first be excluded.

Certain organic conditions may produce symptoms of anxiety. Most commonly thyrotoxicosis, but also hypoglycaemia, Crohn's disease, paroxysmal tachycardia, toxic confusional state, and, rarely, phaeochromocytomas can present in this way.

EFFECTS OF BENZODIAZEPINES

The minor tranquillizers are drugs which diminish feelings of anxiety, tension and panic. In order to avoid confusion with the term 'major tranquillizer' – in other words, neuroleptic (see Chapter 2) – the anxiety-relieving drugs should be called anxiolytics.

All sedative-hypnotics have anxiolytic properties. However, agents such as alcohol, barbiturates and meprobamate relieve anxiety only at doses which produce sleepiness, lethargy and impaired mental activity and coordination. There was not a more selective anxiolytic drug until Sternbach discovered chlordiazepoxide, which was introduced in 1961. This was the first widely used benzodiazepine. The benzodiazepines proved to be powerfully anxiolytic with less sedation than that produced by the older drugs. Nevertheless, large doses are hypnotic and even with anxiolytic doses mental function is impaired, the chance of road traffic accidents being significantly raised.

In addition to anxiety-reducing and sedative properties, the basic actions of the benzodiazepines include muscle relaxation, impairment of learning and accelerated forgetting of learned behaviour, increased appetite and anticonvulsant effects.

Effects of benzodiazepines

- Reduction of anxiety
- Sedation
- Muscle relaxation
- Impairment of learning
- Accelerated forgetting of learned behaviour
- Increased appetite
- Anticonvulsant effects

Toxic effects

The main differences in toxicity between the benzodiazepines and the older hypno-sedatives are that drugs such as the barbiturates are:

1. Powerful depressants of the respiratory and cardiovascular systems.
2. Enzyme inducers, and can thus predispose to drug interactions.
3. Powerful drugs of dependence with physical as well as psychological components to the drug withdrawal state.

On the other hand, the adverse effects of the benzodiazepines can be divided into the following categories:

Dose-dependent CNS actions These include fatigue, weakness, tiredness, somnolence, diplopia, ataxia, slurred speech, motor incoordination, prolonged reaction time, reduced attention span, impaired mental activity.

Unusual idiosyncratic CNS actions These include rage, paradoxical excitement (especially in children), acute confusional state (especially in the elderly), garrulousness, 'drunkenness', atypical antisocial behaviour, hypnagogic hallucinations, Korsakoff-like syndrome, depression, argumentative behaviour.

Respiratory or circulatory collapse Little respiratory or cardiovascular depression occurs even with large doses. However, fatal respiratory or circulatory collapse can result from moderate doses taken with alcohol or other central depressants; and respiratory failure can be produced by benzodiazepines in patients with chronic hypoxic lung disease.

Allergy This is uncommon, but rashes and anaphylaxis can occur.

Low addiction potential Compared with the barbiturates, the benzodiazepines have a low addiction potential. Nevertheless, large doses of the latter, taken for prolonged periods lead to a withdrawal state. This begins two to ten days after stopping the drug and consists of anxiety, restlessness, insomnia and anorexia. Status epilepticus or a delirium tremens-like syndrome can develop.

Enzyme inducers The benzodiazepines are not powerful enzyme-inducing agents and do not usually produce drug interactions by this mechanism. Their central depressant action is greatly increased by the concomitant administration of other sedatives.

Thrombophlebitis When injected intravenously these drugs may produce pain and even thrombophlebitis. Accidental intra-arterial injection is dangerous and can result in arterial spasm and gangrene.

INDIVIDUAL BENZODIAZEPINES

The benzodiazepines can, from a practical point of view, be divided into two groups (see table opposite):

1. Long-acting, mostly with considerable conversion to active metabolites.
2. Shorter-acting, with little or no conversion to active metabolites.

Chlordiazepoxide (Librium)

In the 1930s L. H. Sternbach synthesized a number of heterocyclic dyes while he was working at Cracow University in Poland. After he had transferred to the research division of Hoffman-La Roche Inc in the United States, he produced a large number of chemical derivatives of these substances between 1955 and 1960 in order to produce unique molecules which could be tested for possible tranquillizer activity[11]. There was no rational basis for the choice of these dyestuff derivatives – it was merely that Sternbach had previously gained experience with the compounds and knew he could readily produce new substances from them which could be patented. Many compounds were produced from quinazoline 3-oxides, which were all pharmacologically inactive until he produced a base that was prepared by treating quinazoline *N*-oxide with methylamine. This proved to have remarkable muscular relaxation, sedative and anticonvulsant activity with no effect on the autonomic nervous system or the cardiovascular system (thus differing from chlorpromazine, meprobamate and the barbiturates). There was also a taming effect on wild animals, similar to the neuroleptics, but later studies showed that it had no significant antipsychotic activity but was powerfully anxiolytic.

The compound was the first anxiolytic benzodiazepine introduced into clinical medicine under the trade name Librium. The generic name chlordiazepoxide was later

Drug	Usual oral dose range (mg)	Half-life (hours)	Active metabolites
Long-acting benzodiazepines			
Chlordiazepoxide	10–25	3–30	Desmethylchlordiazepoxide Desmethyldiazepam ($t_{1/2}$ = 100 hours) Oxazepam
Diazepam	2–10	20–50	Desmethyldiazepam ($t_{1/2}$ = 100 hours) Oxazepam
Medazepam	5–15	24	Desmethylmedazepam Desmethyldiazepam ($t_{1/2}$ = 100 hours)
Clorazepate	15–30	30–60	Clorazepate is inactive but is completely metabolized to desmethyldiazepam
Clobazam	10–20	24	*N*-desmethylclobazam
Nitrazepam (mainly used as a hypnotic)	5–10	24 (20–30)	No active major product
Flurazepam (mainly used as a hypnotic)	15–30	2	*N*-hydroethyl flurazepam (short $t_{1/2}$); *N*-desalkyl flurazepam ($t_{1/2}$ = 40–250 hours)
Shorter-acting benzodiazepines			
Oxazepam	15–60	5–20	None
Lorazepam	1–2.5	10–20	None
Triazolam	0.125–0.25	2–4	Hydroxytriazolam ($t_{1/2}$ = 7 hours)
Temazepam	10–30	5–20	No major product
Lormetazepam	0.5–1	10 (up to 14 in elderly)	No active metabolites

generally accepted. Early clinical trials confirmed its anxiolytic properties and revealed no organ-specific toxicity. The main hazards were the consequences of dose-dependent CNS depression such as feelings of tiredness, driving accidents and potentiation of other sedatives. In 1961 occasional paradoxical rage and frequent gain in weight were also noted[11].

Actions Since 1960 strenuous efforts have been made to investigate the mode of action of chlordiazepoxide and its analogues. Recent work has indicated that there may be a benzodiazepine receptor in the brain which has the ability to increase the actions of the inhibitory transmitter gamma-aminobutyric acid (GABA)[11]. The interest in finding such a receptor stems from the possibility that an endogenous anxiolytic agent may exist in the brain which could have an adaptive function in response to stress – in a way analogous to that postulated for the endorphins and encephalins acting on the opiate receptor. No endogenous stimulant of the benzodiazepine receptor has so far been discovered, but antagonists have been found which can promote fits.

GABA effects The highest concentration of the receptor is present in the cerebral cortex and high concentrations exist in the cerebellum and limbic system. Lower density of receptors is measured in the basal ganglia. Relatively few are detected in the brain stem and corpus callosum. These distributions roughly parallel the regions where GABA receptors are found in the brain. GABA is probably the most important inhibitory neurotransmitter in nervous tissue, and the high density of its receptors in the cerebral cortex may reflect a physiological mechanism in preventing excessive spread of nerve impulses relating to muscular activity. It follows that a possible explanation of the anticonvulsant action of the benzodiazepines is potentiation of GABA effects in the motor cortex. Similarly the anxiolytic properties of the group are due to an inhibitory action on the limbic system. The latter is an anatomically diffuse system that includes the ventral tegmental nuclei and amygdala which are concerned with the memory, expression and integration of emotional reactions. The muscle-relaxant effects of the benzodiazepines may be due to enhancement of the actions of inhibitory neurotransmitters in the spinal cord concerned with modulating the activity of the anterior horn cell.

Pharmacokinetics Chlordiazepoxide is well absorbed from the small intestine, but in the elderly absorption is slower than in younger subjects. Peak levels are attained about 1 hour after oral administration. By contrast absorption is greatly delayed following intramuscular administration, the peak appearing at 4–12 hours. In the blood it is 87–88 per cent bound to plasma protein. Tissue binding is not so extensive as with the tricyclic antidepressants, the V_d being 0.35 l/kg.

Chlordiazepoxide is a weak enzyme inducer, but its own metabolism may be accelerated by previous exposure to phenobarbitone, DDT, lynoestrenol and spironolactone.

There is no close correlation between blood levels and clinical effects – but in most subjects profound psychosedation occurs with plasma levels of 5 μg/ml and anxiolytic activity with little sedation at about 0.7 μg/ml plasma.

The terminal half-life varies between 5 – 30 hours in different subjects and tends to rise with age. Active metabolites are produced, the main ones being desmethylchlordiazepoxide, demoxepam and desmethyldiazepam.

The parent drug and its metabolites are excreted mainly in the urine, but some biliary excretion and enterohepatic circulation also occur.

Uses Chlordiazepoxide is mainly administered orally and is used for short-term treatment of anxiety states, panic attacks and restlessness accompanying withdrawal of other sedative drugs and alcohol. The drug is also useful as a premedication for surgical and investigative procedures.

Diazepam

Diazepam was the second major benzodiazepine to be introduced into clinical practice. Although on a weight basis it is more potent than chlordiazepoxide, it has similar pharmacological properties.

Pharmacokinetics Absorption from the gut is complete and the time to peak is 1–4 hours. As with chlordiazepoxide, absorption from an intramuscular injection is slow (time to peak 4–12 hours) and the height of the peak level is reduced. The elimination half-life is 20–50 hours – but this is further prolonged in the elderly. The volume of distribution varies between 0.3 and 1.3 l/kg in young adults. This also rises (up to 2 l/kg) in the elderly. In the newborn – particularly in premature infants – $t_{1/2}\beta$ is also prolonged (40–100 hours) and the volume of distribution is low. In the neonate too the main metabolite is desmethyldiazepam, while from the age of three there are roughly equal amounts of desmethyldiazepam, *N*-methyloxazepam and oxazepam. An entero-hepatic circulation occurs and this may produce a transient increase in blood levels of active metabolites and drug about six hours after a single intravenous dose of diazepam. Because of biliary excretion 9–10 per cent of diazepam and its metabolites appear in the faeces.

As the half-life of desmethyldiazepam (96 hours) is longer than that of diazepam, the former will take longer to reach steady state (five half-lives = twenty days), but during this time cumulation occurs. The metabolites are largely excreted in conjugated form; oxazepam for example is eliminated almost exclusively as the glucuronide.

Diazepam is highly protein bound in the plasma (95–97.5 per cent). In severe hypoalbuminaemia complicating cirrhosis of the liver or the nephrotic syndrome, binding is reduced, but this is probably of little clinical significance. However, in patients with cirrhosis the half-life may be considerably prolonged and the clearance is reduced.

The pattern of fall in plasma levels following an intravenous injection may follow either a two- or three-compartment model. This does not reflect any qualitative interindividual difference in pattern of the drug's bodily disposition, but merely underlines the importance of an extended sampling period.

After a single intravenous dose of 10–20 mg, a peak level of approximately 1 μg/ml is attained. This corresponds to the concentration usually required to produce dysarthria, ptosis, profound psychosedation and anterograde amnesia. Some children and many alcoholics, however, may not be sedated at this plasma level.

Uses In addition to its application in panic attacks and other acute exacerbations of anxiety, diazepam is widely used as a premedication agent before surgical and investigational treatment. Despite its long half-life and extensive conversion to active metabolites some patients find diazepam a perfectly satisfactory hypnotic – certainly on the night before an operation it is very successful in reducing anxious anticipation and thus promoting sleep.

Diazepam has muscle-relaxing properties and may help in painful musculoarticular conditions where there may be a vicious circle of pain causing spasm causing pain. Under these circumstances the drug is given with an analgesic.

Diazepam is available as 2, 5 and 10 mg tablets, 5 and 10 mg suppositories and as injection. The injection is used for rapid effect in status epilepticus, acute anxiety, muscular spasm, and prior to unpleasant procedures. The effect comes on in 60–90 seconds (in other words, much slower than with intravenous barbiturates) and the dose which produces anterograde amnesia and alleviation of anxiety is that which causes ptosis and dysarthria. The dose for this varies greatly, but is usually 2.5–10 mg. The injection is given over 3–5 minutes. Rapid administration – particularly if the patient has previously been given a sedative premedication – can cause transient apnoea. Pain on injection intravenously is very common and this may be followed by thrombophlebitis in about 6 per cent of patients. Accidental intra-arterial injection can produce arterial spasm and this can lead to gangrene. Much of the irritant property of diazepam injection is due to the glycol used to keep the diazepam in solution. An emulsion of diazepam (Diazemuls) is prepared in an oil-in-water emulsion similar to Intralipid. This is injected intravenously and causes a much lower incidence of pain and thrombophlebitis.

Midazolam

Midazolam is the first water-soluble benzodiazepine. At present it is only available in injectable form – the solution being at acid pH. When it is injected intravenously the molecular configuration changes at physiological pH and becomes the highly potent, lipid-soluble benzodiazepine with the typical properties of the group. While in water-soluble form in acid solution, the preparation can be diluted with water.

Pharmacokinetics Midazolam is rapidly metabolized and the terminal half-life usually lies between 1.3 and 2.2 hours. None of the metabolites appear to be active – the principal product is alpha-hydroxy midazolam and this has a $t_{1/2}\beta$ of 1–1½ hours. Unlike diazepam there is no resurgence of action due to enterohepatic circulation.

Actions On intravenous injection the onset of profound sedation or sleep (depending on dose and premedication) is 60–100 seconds. Transient apnoea may occur with large doses (for example, 10 mg given over 1 minute). The elderly appear to be more sensitive to the drug's effects even though the $t_{1/2}\alpha$ may be shorter in such patients.

Amnesia is more frequently produced than with diazepam and may last for up to 1 hour after administration. Recovery is rapid and the patient is usually able to walk without ataxia within 8 hours (compared with 24 for intravenous diazepam).

Use At present the drug is used to produce profound hypnosedation during dental surgery, gastroscopy, endoscopy, cytoscopy and bronchoscopy and cardiac catheterization. It is also being evaluated as an inducing agent for general anaesthesia.

The drug is given intravenously in a dose of approximately 0.07 mg/kg body weight. The injection is carried out slowly until ptosis or dysarthria develop. The usual dose for this in adults is 2.5–10 mg; in the elderly 2.5 mg is usually sufficient. Alcoholics require a sedating premedication, and even then adequate effects sometimes may not be achieved with large doses of benzodiazepines. As the effect may not start for 2 minutes and the peak effect may be delayed for 10 minutes or longer, great care is needed with intravenous benzodiazepines so as not to overdose inadvertently. A slow injection followed by an adequate period of observation is required.

Clobazam

This is a 1,5 benzodiazepine with similar anxiolytic activity to the other 1,4 benzodiazepines, but with less sedative and depressive actions. Motor activity is reduced only on high doses. The usual adult dose is one 10 mg capsule three times a day.

Case history: doing without drugs

A successful director of an advertising firm was referred to hospital because he was found to have tachycardia on a routine medical examination. On examination at the hospital he appeared tense, anxious and hyperkinetic. He had been prescribed diazepam in the past and found that he felt he could not work well when he was even slightly sedated. On questioning he said he often found it difficult to fall asleep at night. A discussion about the possible benefits of relaxation exercises resulted in the patient showing an interest in learning this technique. He became proficient in maintaining muscular relaxation and slow controlled breathing for twenty minutes in bed each night before falling asleep; no more difficulty was experienced with sleeping. After two months he found that he could successfully apply relaxation techniques at work when an anxiety-provoking situation arose.

Case history: successful use of diazepam

Mr N. is a successful retail salesman of woollen garments. He consulted his physician because of attacks of sweating, shaking and fear. These did not occur at work but during recreation – typically when going to his pub or golf club, and the attacks were so severe that he always had to return home. Previously lorazepam 1 mg three times a day did not prevent these episodes. He expressed an interest in relaxation techniques and enjoyed reading about these. The attacks persisted, however, so he was advised to take diazepam 2 mg at the onset of attacks, and this proved almost invariably successful in terminating the episodes of panic within twenty to thirty minutes. However, he found it inconvenient not to be able to drive after he took his tablet.

METABOLIC INTERRELATIONSHIPS OF SOME BENZODIAZEPINES

Chlorazepate is not itself absorbed but is converted in an acid environment to desmethyldiazepam (nordiazepam). This hydrolytic step normally occurs in the stomach.

If gastric acidity is reduced by antacid therapy, the rate but not the extent of the conversion is reduced. According to current jargon chlorazepate is thus acting as a prodrug.

Prazepam, demoxepam and medazepam are also converted to desmethyldiazepam (nordiazepam). The latter clearly plays a central role in the metabolic interconversions of the benzodiazepines:

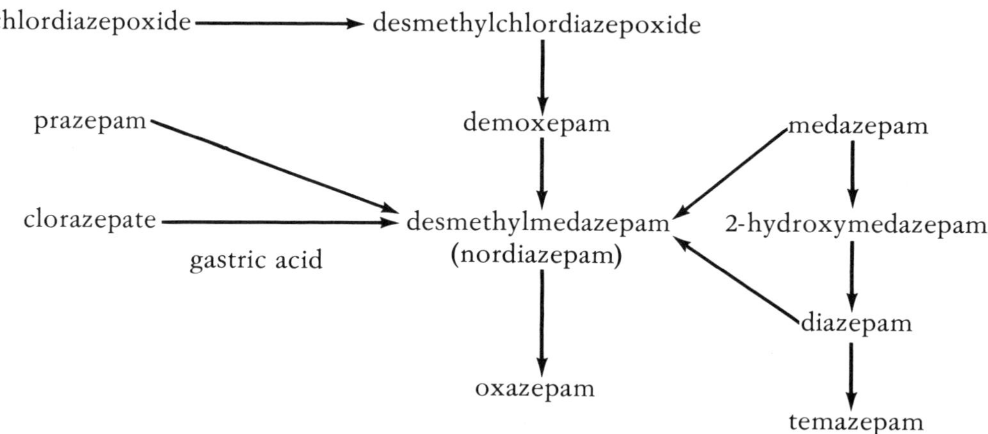

Temazepam is mainly excreted unchanged apart from conjugation to its glucuronide. The latter has a shorter $t_{1/2}$ than the parent drug and produces a briefer period of sedation.

PRACTICAL POINTS

- Behavioural and supportive treatment is essential in all patients with agoraphobia. Severe, chronic, intractable agoraphobia may respond to tricyclic or MAOI antidepressant drugs (see Chapter 3).
- Relaxation exercises and cognitive therapy can be successful in anxiety states.
- Anxiolytics can be used for panic attacks but not for long-term treatment.
- The benzodiazepines have a relatively low dependence potential, but dependence can occur and there are various other adverse side-effects.

5
Drugs used in organic brain disease

BACKGROUND

At present there is no convincing evidence that drug treatment can influence the progress of the common forms of chronic organic brain disease. Nevertheless, dementia due to Alzheimer's disease and to vascular occlusion is very common, affecting around 10 per cent of people over seventy. Thus even a modest reduction in disability could produce a startling improvement in the overall wellbeing of the older members of the population. It is because of this that much research effort is being expended in examining the actions of new compounds on the dementias of later life.

MANAGEMENT OF DEMENTIA

Blood flow through the brain represents a large proportion of the cardiac output, and oxygen consumption by brain is about one-quarter of that of the body. Cerebral blood flow increases with mental and physical activity and with sensory stimulation. This is at least partly due to the increased production of carbon dioxide and acid metabolites – all of which are vasodilators. Hypoxia also increases cerebral blood flow. In addition, carotid chemoreceptors and baroreceptors influence flow reflexly, probably by sympathetic vasoconstrictor nerve fibres which directly supply cerebral vessels.

Blood flow to the brain progressively decreases with age after early adult life. This is mainly secondary to alterations in brain neurones, which result in reduced metabolic requirements. In addition, degenerative occlusive vascular disease may make a smaller contribution to this decline.

Alzheimer's disease and multi-infarct dementia

In senile dementia, 50–75 per cent of patients are suffering from primary neuronal degeneration (Alzheimer's dementia). Vascular disease (multi-infarct dementia) accounts for 10–20 per cent of cases. However, before attempting any treatment it is necessary to ensure that the patient does not suffer from a reversible syndrome such as drug intoxication (in particular hypnosedative and antiparkinsonian anticholinergic drugs), infection, anaemia, myxoedema or other metabolic disturbance. Depression can also produce a confusional state. It has been estimated that 10–20 per cent of patients with dementia have a reversible underlying cause[12].

In Alzheimer's disease, in which the cerebral blood flow is reduced secondary to neuronal degeneration, there is a normal cerebral vasodilator response to carbon dioxide, while in multi-farct dementia there is a considerable reduction in cerebral blood flow and an impaired vascular response to carbon dioxide.

Intracerebral steal In this condition, the use of cerebral vasodilators can result in decreased blood flow in the diseased areas because of localized dilatation in the healthy parts of the brain. This is called 'intracerebral steal' and is due to a combination of blood vessel occlusion, surrounding vasodilatation and lack of vascular reactivity in the ischaemic areas. It is therefore not surprising that cerebral vasodilators have proved disappointing in Alzheimer's disease and in ischaemic dementia. However, the vasodilators which have an additional action on cerebral metabolism (such as dihydroergotoxine and naftidrofuryl, see pages 76–7) do seem to produce a small but significant improvement in memory and behaviour.

The role of drug treatment in dementia

Thus it appears that drug treatment plays only a minor part in the management of dementia. The main therapeutic effort should be with the patient and his family, and should deal with interpersonal, social and practical difficulties. Nevertheless if depression develops, antidepressant drugs may provide relief, and, similarly, anxiolytic drugs may assist in the management of an anxiety crisis. Episodes of agitation and confusion generally respond to neuroleptics. Thioridazine (see page 22) is widely used in senile dementia for this purpose. Initially an oral dose of 10 mg 8-hourly is used, and the dose is slowly increased if necessary. Prolonged treatment with thioridazine is less often associated with extrapyramidal toxicity than with chlorpromazine, perphenazine or trifluoperazine. However, orthostatic hypotension may predispose to falls.

But even with specific psychiatric syndromes arising in a patient suffering from dementia, supportive treatment is of extreme importance. Frequent personal contact and maintaining a supportive, warm and caring environment are much more effective than drugs. The patient must be encouraged to go on learning physical skills (such as balance), coming in contact with the arts and keeping in touch with everyday life (such as political events and current fashions in thought). Memory is not usually destroyed in the dementias, but learning is slowed and more prolonged exposure to new facts is required. This must be encouraged.

Case history: organic versus non-organic mental illness (1)

Fifty-two-year-old housewife, Mrs J. W., married mother of two, was admitted to hospital following several months of erratic behaviour. On admission she was confused, disorientated for time and place, and showed a tendency to wander off the ward. Psychological testing showed gross impairment, and a diagnosis of presenile dementia was made. Her sleep was disturbed, she was particularly restless at night and she required neuroleptic medication.

Detailed investigation failed to offer a cause of the dementing process and a CAT brain scan showed no abnormality. A senior psychiatrist was consulted about this patient and he considered that she could be suffering from an atypical depressive illness which mimicked some of the features of dementia. She was thus vigorously treated with antidepressant medication, in this instance clomipramine 150 mg at night and tryptophan 1 g daily, and made a dramatic recovery. Her intellectual and cognitive functions on repeat testing after treatment were completely normal.

This case highlights the occasional difficulty in clearly identifying a depressive illness. Depressive 'pseudodementia' usually has clinical features of depression which alert the clinician to the underlying illness, although in this case it was difficult to make a correct diagnostic formulation until a CAT scan and a wider range of special investigations had excluded organic brain disease. The addition of tryptophan to clomipramine in the patient's treatment is an attempt both to increase the amount of available tryptophan in the brain as well as to increase production of the relevant neurotransmitter at the synaptic site. Tryptophan is not very useful as an antidepressant in its own right (see page 56).

Case history: organic versus non-organic mental illness (2)

Seventy-year-old Mrs P. presented with hallucinations, both visual and auditory, and a delusion that her neighbours were trying to poison her. These symptoms had been present for approximately a week. She was medicated with a neuroleptic (in this case, thioridazine 50 mg) but remained confused and distressed, requiring admission. Once in hospital, and receiving no medication, she improved rapidly, all symptoms abating.

When her medication was stopped, however, she developed parkinsonism. It later emerged that she had previously been started on levodopa for Parkinson's disease by her own doctor, and it appeared that the drug had precipitated a psychotic episode. Levodopa and related drugs may cause a toxic confusional state, or a state mimicking schizophrenia in patients with spontaneous Parkinson's disease.

Up to 16 per cent of hospital admissions to psychogeriatric units are due directly to medication. These effects may be caused by the drugs themselves, given in excessive doses, or secondary drug effects such as hypotension, injuries from falls and chest infections, or paradoxical responses to the drug itself, such as disinhibition or excitability following certain sedative-hypnotics.

DRUG TREATMENT OF OTHER TYPES OF ORGANIC BRAIN DISEASE

Acute stroke

Following an acute cerebral infarction there is decreased blood flow in the lesion and a surrounding zone of increased blood flow. The area in which the infarction is developing shows a reduced or abolished response to vasodilator drugs and to carbon dioxide.

Because the response to vasodilators is normal in the surrounding brain tissue, such drugs as papaverine or betahistine can lead to the 'intracerebral steal' phenomenon and in this way further reduce the perfusion of the diseased region.

Chronic stroke

Cerebral reactivity gradually returns between one to six weeks following acute ischaemia in a region of the brain. After this time some increase in blood flow in the diseased region can be induced by papaverine. Nevertheless this does not appear to be accompanied by any functional improvement in the neurological condition.

Transient ischaemic attacks (little strokes)

Short-lived episodes of focal cerebral ischaemia are often associated with carotid artery degenerative disease and are probably usually due to small emboli arising in the heart or carotid vessels. The attacks usually resolve within several hours.

Vasodilators do not prevent or shorten the attacks. Drug treatment is not usually helpful but drugs which inhibit platelet aggregation and anticoagulants may reduce the chances of recurrence.

Drugs influencing the progress of common forms of chronic organic brain disease, including dementia, can be divided into three groups:

- Vasodilators
- Metabolic precursors and modifiers
- Anticoagulants and platelet antiaggregants.

VASODILATORS ACTING ON THE SYMPATHETIC SYSTEM

Ergot derivatives

Dihydroergotoxine mesylate is a mixture of the methane sulphonates of dihydrogenated ergocornine, ergocristine and ergocryptine. Ergot derivatives of this family are alpha-receptor blockers and have a direct vasoconstrictor activity. Dihydrogenation abolishes the vasoconstrictor activity, thus unmasking the alpha-blocking effects (which reduce sympathetic vasoconstrictor tone). Dihydroergotoxine mesylate has weak dopamine agonist and emetic properties. In addition, it decreases the brain's oxygen requirements by inhibiting the breakdown of adenosine triphosphate (ATP) and by blocking the action of phosphodiesterase. The latter action also contributes to vasodilator actions. Although the substance is a vasodilator, it does not appear to increase cerebral blood flow.

Dose and effects The usual oral dose is 4.5 mg daily. Toxic effects are buccal irritation, nausea, postural hypotension, sinus bradycardia, nasal stuffiness and rashes. Peak blood levels are attained at 2–3 hours and the elimination half-life is approximately 12 hours. If toxicity is severe at the time of peak absorption, the dose may be divided during the day.

In a number of trials in elderly demented patients there has been some improvement in cognitive function and walking, and reduction in confusion[13]. Improvement, however, takes three weeks to start.

Isoxsuprine

This substance is a vasodilator which also reduces blood viscosity and inhibits platelet aggregation. Vasodilatation is by alpha-receptor blockade, beta-receptor stimulation and by inhibition of adenylcyclase. Cerebral blood flow is not increased.

Dose and effects The oral dose of the sustained release capsules is 20 mg 6-hourly or 40 mg twice daily. Toxicity includes flushing, palpitations and postural hypotension.

In patients with dementia, some trials have demonstrated an improvement in cognitive function[13]. Possible benefit could develop in peripheral vascular disease. Nylidrin is a similar drug to isoxsuprine.

VASODILATORS ON THE BLOOD VESSEL WALL

Cyclandelate

This drug relaxes vascular smooth muscle and in this way produces generalized vasodilatation. In some, but not all, studies in patients with cerebrovascular disease an increase in cerebral blood flow has been demonstrated. Cyclandelate may possibly increase cerebral glucose utilization and increase the resistance of the brain to hypoxia.

Dose and effects The oral daily dose is 1.2–1.6 g, given in divided amounts. Toxic actions are not usually severe; dyspepsia, flushing, palpitations and headache may occur.

As with all drugs in the treatment of dementia, the results of clinical trials vary, but a number of investigations have shown an improvement in psychomotor performance and an arrest of progressive intellectual and social deterioration[13].

Naftidrofuryl

Naftidrofuryl had direct smooth muscle-relaxing and weak ganglion-blocking effects. Experimental studies show an increase in glucose utilization and raised intracellular levels of ATP, which suggest a possible protective action against tissue hypoxia and ischaemia. In human subjects acceleration of glycolysis has also been demonstrated.

No increase in cerebral blood flow has been produced by naftidrofuryl[13].

Dose and effects The oral dose is 100–200 mg 8-hourly. Toxicity is similar to that produced by cyclandelate: dyspepsia, flushing, headaches, palpitations; there may also be diarrhoea and insomnia. The drug is well absorbed from the intestine but has a short half-life (forty minutes).

Several controlled and uncontrolled clinical trials on patients with cerebrovascular disease and dementia have revealed an improvement in mental function and memory with a possible increase in physical activity[13].

Papaverine

This is a non-opioid alkaloid derived from opium. Dioxyline phosphate is a synthetic analogue with similar properties. Papaverine is a relaxer of smooth muscle by direct actions, partly because of inhibition of adenylcyclase. Consistent and significant increases in cerebral blood flow are produced in normal subjects and in patients with chronic cerebrovascular disease.

Dose and effects Papaverine is given orally as sustained release capsules in doses of 150–300 mg 12-hourly; dioxyline phosphate is given orally in doses of 100–400 mg 8-hourly. The elimination half-life of papaverine is 0.5–2 hours and its action on cerebral blood flow is short-lived. Toxicity includes drowsiness, giddiness and constipation. The action of levodopa in Parkinson's disease may be antagonized.

OTHER TYPES OF VASODILATORS

Nicotinic acid and nicotinamide

Nicotinic acid and nicotinyl alcohol have identical vasodilator actions. Tetranicotinoyl fructose is broken down in the intestine to nicotinic acid and fructose. Inositol hexanicotinate has identical actions to nicotinic acid. Nicotinic acid is converted in the body to nicotinamide. Nicotinic acid produces widespread vasodilatation. It also lowers plasma fibrinogen, cholesterol and triglycerides in doses which produce facial flushing and paraesthesiae.

Dose and effects In the treatment of hypercholesterolaemia 1–6 g of nicotinic acid are given daily in divided doses. In some patients indomethacin reduces flushing of the skin. No convincing effects have been demonstrated on cerebral blood flow or cerebrovascular disease.

Betahistine

This is an analogue of histamine which stimulates only H_1 receptors. It is an effective cerebral vasodilator.

Dose and effects The oral dose is 8–16 mg 8-hourly; nausea, headache and flushing may develop.

In patients with multi-infarct dementia and vertebrobasilar insufficiency significant improvement has been measured in several independent trials[13].

METABOLIC PRECURSORS AND MODIFIERS

Several drugs (apart from some of the vasodilators) influence brain metabolism.

Pentifylline and meclofenoxate

The former is a nicotinic acid conjugate of a caffeine derivative which possibly increases the ability of brain neurones to utilize glucose. Meclofenoxate reduces oxygen uptake by the brain.

Deanol (2-dimethylaminoethanol)

This is a precursor of choline. Although claims have been made that deanol improves memory and acts as a mental energizer in dementia, this has not been subject to a double-blind trial. There is, however, evidence that inhibitors of the cholinergic system – such as atropine and benzhexol – impair memory, while acetylcholine agonists and choline may improve normal memory. In patients with Alzheimer's disease physostigmine and arecholine may possibly improve short-term visual memory.

ANTICOAGULANTS AND PLATELET ANTIAGGREGANTS

This group of drugs is used for the prophylaxis of thromboembolic disease. In patients suffering from transient ischaemic attacks, the chance of developing a completed stroke is reduced by the administration of the anticoagulant warfarin. The drug is usually continued for one year, controlling the daily dose by repeated estimations of the prothrombin time.

If a cerebral embolus has arisen in a patient with atrial fibrillation, then initially drug control of the arrhythmia is attempted. If sinus rhythm is not attained, then prolonged use of an oral anticoagulant, such as warfarin, is considered. Anticoagulants are dangerous drugs because of the risk of bleeding; because of this, drugs which modify platelet function are commonly used.

Transient ischaemic attacks can occur due to emboli arising on atheromatous plaques. The initial event in the formation of such emboli is the adhesion of blood platelets to the abnormal vascular intima. This causes the release of thromboxanes which are powerful platelet aggregants. The resulting platelet thrombus forms the nucleus of a blood clot. Drugs which inhibit platelet stickiness also inhibit platelet adherence to the vessel wall and prevent the formation of platelet thrombi. The following drugs are used to modify platelet function in this way:

- Aspirin
- Sulphinpyrazone
- Dipyridamole

Aspirin

The Boston Collaborative Drug Surveillance Program showed that recurrence of myocardial infarction was less frequent in patients who regularly took aspirin[14]. Since then trials have suggested that aspirin reduces the incidence of cerebral ischaemic attacks[15]. About 30 per cent of patients with these attacks develop a stroke within three years and it has been suggested that aspirin may (like anticoagulants) reduce this risk[15].

Dose and effects The dose of aspirin for optimum antiaggregation activity has not been established, and in various trials ranges from about 300 mg twice weekly to 1 g daily. A middle-of-the-road suggestion is 300 mg daily[14]. Much of the toxicity of aspirin is dose-dependent, and therefore at the suggested dose toxicity should not be a major problem. Nevertheless, patients with active peptic ulceration and atopic asthma may experience adverse effects. Aspirin is contraindicated in patients taking anti-coagulants.

Sulphinpyrazone

Although sulphinpyrazone decreases the fragility of platelets, thus inhibiting the release of thromboxanes, there is no evidence that the drug prevents thrombolic and embolic cerebral disease. However, the drug is active in preventing thrombosis in patients with prosthetic heart valves and arteriovenous shunts, and may have some value in secondary prevention of myocardial infarction.

Dose and effects The dose is 400 mg twice daily. Toxicity is unusual, but there may be dyspepsia.

Dipyridamole

This drug was originally used as a coronary artery vasodilator. However, it also reduces platelet aggregation. It is effective in decreasing embolus formation when used with anticoagulants in patients with prosthetic heart valves. In cerebrovascular disease there is little evidence that it has prophylactic activity.

Dose and effects Dipyridamole with aspirin may have some value in preventing fatal reinfarction within 6 months of a myocardial infarct. The oral dose is 400 mg daily. Headache and nausea may result from this dose.

PRACTICAL POINTS

- Drug treatment plays only a minor role in the management of dementia, the main therapy being to deal with the patient's interpersonal, social and practical problems.
- Exclude treatable causes of dementia such as mental disorders due to drugs – in particular withdraw all sedatives in elderly patients who present with confusional episodes. Sixty per cent of brain tumours present as psychiatric illness.
- Acute delirium can be ameliorated with benzodiazepines. Neuroleptics are also effective but can provoke fits, particularly in alcoholics.
- Recent trials have indicated that aspirin can reduce the incidence of cerebral ischaemic attacks.

6
The management of sleep disturbance

BACKGROUND

The exact nature of sleep and its physiological function are not understood. One hypothesis is that sleep is restorative and nutritive[16]. Such ideas arose from the observations of surges in growth hormone release and increases in cerebral blood flow during sleep.

There is wide interindividual variation in the pattern of sleep and in total sleep requirement. In general, sleep can be divided into orthodox or non-rapid eye movement (NREM) sleep – which accounts for approximately 80 per cent of total sleep time – and paradoxical or rapid eye movement (REM) sleep. It is during paradoxical sleep that vivid dreaming is most often described, and it is the relationship of paradoxical to orthodox sleep cycles that seems to affect total sleep requirements.

Hypnotic drugs influence both types of sleep, but paradoxical sleep is more strikingly suppressed. On withdrawal of the hypnotic there is a rebound increase in paradoxical sleep which corresponds clinically to nightmares and repeated awakenings, and occasionally atypical delirious states occur, analogous to delirium tremens or

Figure 8 Dreaming rebound on withdrawal of barbiturates.

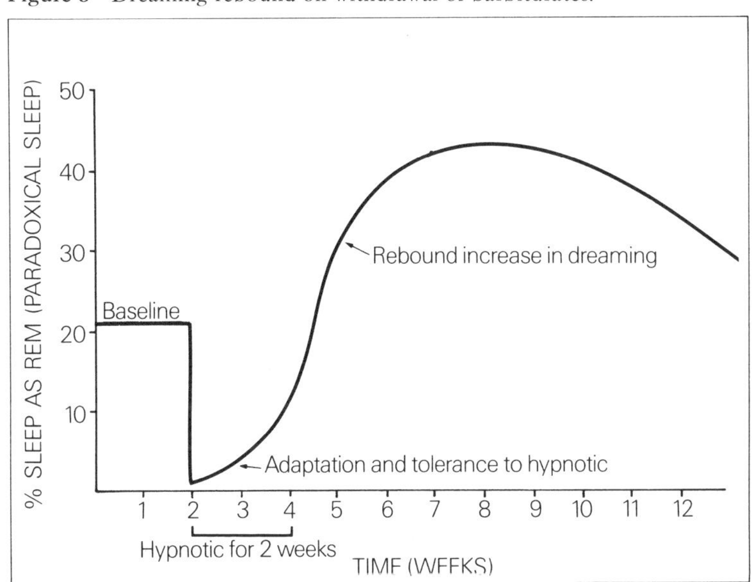

alcohol withdrawal. Tricyclic antidepressants suppress paradoxical sleep initially, but once tolerance develops, sleep patterns return to normal. Monoamine oxidase inhibitors (MAOIs) abolish paradoxical sleep totally for the duration of treatment. Sedative antidepressant drugs have an effect on sleep which is a useful adjunct in the treatment of many depressed patients; however they occupy little place in the treatment of primary sleep disorders.

INSOMNIA

A classification of sleep disorders is as follows:

- **Primary**
- **Secondary**
  - Physiological
  - Pathological
  - Environmental

Primary

Some healthy individuals suffer severe insomnia for no apparent reason. This group needs to be managed with particular caution because indiscriminate use of hypnotics can readily lead to drug dependence.

Secondary

Physiological Changes in sleep rhythms can produce temporary sleep difficulties, as seen, for example, in shift workers and aircrews.

Pathological This large group includes both psychological and physical disorders. Sleep disturbances may be a feature of psychiatric disorders such as depressive illness, anxiety states, schizophrenia and emotional stress reactions. Those dependent on hypnotics or alcohol frequently suffer from sleep problems. Beta-blocking drugs can cause nightmares. Disturbed sleep can also result from such physical conditions as breathlessness, cough, pain, itching and a full bladder or rectum.

Environmental A cold bedroom, stimulant beverages and noise are important and correctable causes of insomnia. A restless or loudly snoring nocturnal partner may cause more difficulties.

Initial management of insomnia

1. Look for treatable underlying conditions. This may involve using appropriate drugs to treat left ventricular failure, bronchospasm or pain. Prostatic hypertrophy may necessitate referral to a genitourinary surgeon.
2. Advise that tea and coffee may have to be avoided during the last five hours before going to bed.
3. Hypnotics should not normally be prescribed in the initial treatment of depression.

4. In all patients with secondary insomnia the use of hypnotics may be avoided by reassuring that the sleep problem will go once the underlying situation has resolved.

Insomnia in the elderly

Insomnia in the elderly poses particular problems. There is a normal reduction in sleep requirement in ageing. Not only is hypnotic therapy often inappropriate, but may produce considerable harm; as a group, the elderly are particularly susceptible to the toxic effects of sedatives. Iatrogenic problems account for up to 20 per cent of admissions to psychogeriatric units.

More insidious is the hangover effect experienced by this large and increasing population group. Even when hypnotics have produced a good night's sleep, this is at the cost of impairment of mental and social functioning during the next day. The newer short-acting hypnotics have been developed in order to reduce this hangover effect. One of the studies on nitrazepam indicates that elderly people suffering from the effects of overmedication with this drug do not complain and do not even realize that there may be a drug problem[16]. Such drug-induced deterioration in physical and mental wellbeing frequently goes unnoticed for long periods. Certainly if a hypnotic is prescribed for a patient in this age group, the choice must be particularly carefully made and the lowest effective dose used for the minimum period.

The pressure on the practitioner to prescribe is great and the expectation of patients is high. A busy surgery often lowers the tolerance to prescribing, and hypnotics are probably the drugs most often left for a patient to collect as a 'repeat' without further consultation with the doctor.

The development of tolerance to hypnotics underlines the need to avoid the long-term use of a night sedative.

Suggested management of insomnia

Alteration of presleep behaviour Daytime napping should be cut down to a minimum and, ideally, avoided altogether. Exercise should be encouraged. Few patients will carry out a graded exercise programme, but gardening, shopping, housework and using stairs instead of lifts may be an effective substitute.

For most people a warm bath has a pleasant relaxing effect. Many find that sexual activity has the same result.

Unrealistic expectations are often encountered. It is not unusual to find patients retiring early in the evening and expecting nine or ten hours sleep. Reading for one or two of those hours before bed may be preferable.

Alteration of environment Neither an uncomfortable bed, a noisy room nor a disturbing partner are conducive to a good night's sleep, particularly in those people who would describe themselves as 'light sleepers' (and are often no different from the vast majority). At the risk of being accused of breaking up relationships, not everyone is suited to a double bed, and two single mattresses – perhaps of the 'zipped-and-linked' type – are often a simple solution to a troublesome situation.

Alteration of underlying problems Anxiety, both acute and chronic, are associated with difficulty in getting off to sleep.

Non-chemical relaxation techniques may prove useful and are available on cassette for use by the patient in the home.

Removal or relief of physical problems are associated with improved sleep, and it is worth remembering that hypnotics are not analgesic and many in fact are hyperalgesic.

Some functional psychiatric disorders (in particular depression and anxiety) are often associated with sleep disturbances and resolution of an episode commonly results in improved sleep patterns.

Diet A heavy meal – particularly one rich in fat – taken within six hours of going to bed may disturb sleep. Alcohol is initially sedating, but when it has been metabolized by the body rebound anxiety, nightmares or insomnia frequently occur.

Commercially available milk-cereal beverages have been shown to prolong total sleep time in those who are accustomed to drinking them before going to bed[16]. Their mode of action is not known, but their most striking effect is in the latter half of the night, during which episodes of waking are reduced in number. These actions seem to be most prominent in the elderly. Tolerance does not develop – in fact the effectiveness of such drinks improves with chronic use.

Tea and coffee, by contrast, can produce sleep disturbances both by cerebral stimulation and by their diuretic actions.

HYPNOTICS

Hypnotics are drugs which produce a state similar to physiological sleep. However, when sleep is drug-induced several abnormalities can be detected, including rapid EEG patterns, suppression of dreaming (paradoxical sleep) and of deep (slow-wave or orthodox) sleep. During dreaming there is an increase in cerebral blood flow and acceleration in protein synthesis in the brain; slow-wave sleep is accompanied by secretion of anabolic hormones and increase in somatic protein synthesis. These are inhibited by hypnotic drugs.

Insomnia is also a common problem (see previously). In a survey carried out in two Scottish cities, 45 per cent of women and 15 per cent of men over forty-five years regularly took hypnotics[16]. These figures are a reflection of patients' assessments of their sleep needs and are not an index of a true physiological requirement.

The most widely used hypnotics are listed opposite above, but not all of these drugs can be recommended for this purpose.

General problems associated with hypnotic use

Initial problems During the first week or two of hypnotic administration the patient often greatly appreciates the ease of falling asleep, suppression of dreaming, lack of nocturnal awakening and prolongation of sleeping time. He feels something substantial has been accomplished.

Recommended for use as hypnotics

- Benzodiazepines
- Chlormethiazole
- Chloral derivatives

Not recommended for use as hypnotics

- Barbiturates
- Piperidinediones (e.g. glutethimide)
- Antihistamines (e.g. promethazine)
- Alcohols (e.g. ethchlorvynol, ethanol)
- Quinazolines (methaqualone)

PROBLEMS WITH HYPNOTIC DRUGS NOT RECOMMENDED FOR USE

Drug	Problems			
	Enzyme induction	CVS and respiratory depression	Dependence	Other
Barbiturates	+++	+++	+++	Paradoxical excitement; confusion in the elderly; rebound CNS hyper-excitability; severe with-drawal problems
Glutethimide	++	+++	+++	Cerebral oedema; anti-cholinergic effect; rebound CNS hyperexcitability
Promethazine	?	+++	?	Great variability in response; vertigo, delirium, excitement, anticholinergic effects
Alcohols				
ethyl alcohol	+	+++	+++	CNS and other organ damage; delirium tremens, etc.
ethchlorvynol	+	+++	+++	Delirium tremens; dizziness, nausea; long $t_{1/2}$ (24 hours)
Methaqualone	Similar in toxicity to barbiturates			

KEY: + mild, ++ moderate, +++ considerable

These benefits, however, are short-lived. Dreaming and repeated awakening return and the sleeping time becomes progressively shorter even though the drug is continued. At this stage there is a temptation to increase the dose; in other words, tolerance has developed. If the patient stops the drug there is immediate difficulty in falling asleep (usually worse than before starting treatment) and sleep is disturbed by frequent, vivid and alarming dreams. In addition, feelings of anxiety become increased and may contribute to the sleep difficulty. This is due to drug dependence and is an expression of physical and psychological withdrawal. There is every incentive for the patient to ask to be put back on his sleeping tablets.

Withdrawal symptoms Even more severe withdrawal states may develop, such as panic attacks and convulsions.

Serious problems The majority of hypnotics are powerful depressors of the respiratory and cardiovascular systems. Suicide and accidental fatal overdose readily happen, particularly if alcohol is taken at about the same time.

Nocturnal confusion One of the commonest causes of nocturnal confusion is the use of hypnotics. Sedative drugs can produce disorientation for time, place and person; delusions of persecution; anxiety and frightening visual hallucinations. After such episodes there is usually no recall of the events during the confusional state. Many elderly patients who become excited and disorientated at night are restored to normality by stopping their night sedative (see Chapter 5). Increasing the dose or variety of sedatives used only aggravates the problem.

'Hangovers' Hangover follows sleep induced by all hypnotics. This may consist of subjective feelings of 'heaviness' or 'muzziness' on awakening, but objective tests show highly significant impairment of mental acuity and reaction time well into the following day[17]. The patients may be ataxic and show other evidence of incoordination. The risk of a driving accident is increased.

Adverse interactions with other drugs Apart from the general property of potentiation of all hypnotics by alcohol, many of these drugs can produce adverse interactions with other drugs. For example, barbiturates and glutethimide are enzyme-inducers and can, in this way, decrease the actions of warfarin, the contraceptive pill, and of steroids, doses of which may have to be readjusted. Chloral hydrate can increase the activity of warfarin by removing the anticoagulant from protein-binding sites in the plasma.

INDIVIDUAL HYPNOTICS RECOMMENDED FOR USE

Benzodiazepines

These are the drugs of choice for sleep induction (see page 67).

The advantages of the benzodiazepines over the older hypnotics is that respiratory depression is slight and the potential for dependence is reduced. Nevertheless, in patients with chronic lung disease (particularly chronic bronchitis and emphysema) fatal respiratory depression may result. Alcohol taken with a benzodiazepine can also cause a fatal outcome.

Nocturnal confusion in the elderly may develop, but this is less serious than with the barbiturates and glutethimide.

Doses and effects Although the benzodiazepines may produce less disturbance of physiological sleep patterns than other hypnotics, the hangover they produce is, if anything, more prolonged as many have long half-lives and some produce long-lived active metabolites. However, some of the newer members of this series (such as temazepam and lormetazepam) have a shorter action and produce no active metabolites (see table of benzodiazepines on page 67).

Total sleeping time does not correspond to blood levels of benzodiazepines, and even long-acting drugs such as diazepam may act as satisfactory hypnotics.

Toxicity of the benzodiazepines is mainly dose-dependent CNS depression. In some patients weakness or ataxia may be produced instead of sedation. Paradoxical excitement, drunken garrulousness and rage are unusual effects. Allergic reactions (including anaphylaxis) do occur but less commonly than with chloral and the other older hypnotics.

These drugs do not produce enzyme induction to a clinically significant degree.

Suicide by benzodiazepine overdose will not be successful unless another central nervous system depressant (such as alcohol) has been taken as well.

Chlormethiazole

This drug has, in recent years, gained popular acceptance as a hypnotic, particularly in geriatric practice and in alcoholics undergoing withdrawal therapy. It is said to produce little or no confusion in the elderly[18].

Chlormethiazole is short-lived in the body. It has a plasma half-life of one hour and is extensively metabolized by the liver. In liver disease considerable reductions in dose are essential.

Dose and effects The usual evening dose is 400 mg. Toxic effects are:

- Nasal, conjunctival and bronchial discomfort before sedation has begun
- Gastric irritation
- Respiratory and cardiovascular depression
- Dependence.

Chlormethiazole produces dependence and is recommended for use in drug withdrawal (including alcohol) and as a hypnotic in organic states in the elderly.

Chloral hydrate

This agent has been used for many years and still appears to be a reasonably safe and effective hypnotic. Serious degrees of dependence are uncommon, but it is a gastric irritant and rashes are common. It can be used in all age groups, including young children.

Chloral is converted to a hydrate in solution. In solid form (such as when combined with phenazone) it appears to produce less gastric irritation than when in solution. Both forms are rapidly absorbed. In the liver an active metabolite, trichlorethanol, is formed. Chloral is rapidly metabolized but trichlorethanol has a half-life of eight hours.

Dose and effects Doses and toxicity of chloral hydrate are shown below.

Derivation	Dose	Preparations
Chloral hydrate	0.5–2.0 g (adult) 30–50 mg/kg (child)	Chloral mixture 500 mg/5 ml; paediatric chloral elixir 200 mg/5 ml; Noctec is a capsule containing 500 mg
Dichloralphenazone	1.2–1.95 g (adult)	Welldorm tablets contain 650 mg; Welldorm elixir 225 mg/5 ml.

Toxic effects of chloral hydrate

- Respiratory and CVS depression
- Gastric irritation
- Rashes: erythematous, scarlatiniform, urticarial, scaling
- Jaundice
- Proteinuria
- Interactions: alcohol ('Mickey Finn'), warfarin

DRUG THERAPY

From a practical prescribing point of view, it is clear that the general public benefits from an educational and hierarchical approach, and that if hypnotics are eventually introduced it should be as part of a treatment programme with aims, goals and a time limit.

A large number of hypnotic agents has been mentioned above. It is clear that most of these are powerful hypnotics. As is true with so many psychotropic drugs, the most effective drugs often have unwanted effects which make their use potentially dangerous. Having said this, there is no reason why anyone who requires an hypnotic should be denied one – with the emphasis on *require* rather than request.

It is ironic that patients often develop a dependence on their hypnotics for a good night's sleep as rapidly as their bodies become tolerant to the drugs and their sleep patterns return to normal.

A case can be made for a verbal contract whereby terms of the treatment are spelled out and agreed upon by both physician and patient. This will have the effect both of clarifying patient expectation and avoiding prolonged exposure to hypnotics with the development of tolerance.

Choice of hypnotic

This is important, and it is now widely accepted that barbiturates and substances with similar qualities, such as meprobamate, should not be used. This is because of the part they play in drug abuse, as well as the difficulty in withdrawal with the development of fits.

The benzodiazepines have a low toxic potential, are relatively safe in overdose (unless in combination with other sedatives), and the newer drugs with a shorter half-life, such as temazepam and lormetazepam, do not generally contribute to a hangover effect in the morning. Nevertheless, prescriptions for benzodiazepines have reached epidemic proportions, and a large number of these could be avoided.

Chlormethiazole, though an effective hypnotic, has been implicated in drug dependence, and its use should be confined to drug and alcohol withdrawal, and in geriatric patients for the treatment of insomnia complicated by behavioural disturbances. Chlormezanone is an alternative to chlormethiazole and is used in doses of 200–400 mg at night for the short-term treatment of insomnia. It is contraindicated in significant hepatic or renal insufficiency. It has muscle relaxant properties.

The oldest hypnotic still in common use today is chloral hydrate and its derivatives. Some side-effects might prove problematic, particularly an unpleasant smell, but it is among the safest agents, and is considered by many as the hypnotic of first choice, particularly in the elderly.

PRACTICAL POINTS

- Insomnia is commonly an expression of reduced physical need for sleep.
- Other causes of insomnia, such as unfavourable environmental conditions and physical illness, may be amenable to correction.
- If a hypnotic is to be used, this should be for limited periods only.
- The barbiturates, glutethimide and similar drugs are not recommended as hypnotics.
- Benzodiazepines are the hypnotics of choice but some physicians also use chloral hydrate or chlormethiazole.
- There is no obvious difference in sleeping time between diazepam (2–5 mg) and benzodiazepines with short half-lives such as triazolam (0.125–0.25 mg), although the latter may produce less hangover.
- Withdrawal symptoms, nocturnal confusion, hangovers and adverse reactions with other drugs are all problems involved with the use of hypnotics
- Relaxation exercises are excellent for the treatment of insomnia due to tension and anxiety.

7
Drug dependence and drug abuse

BACKGROUND

The terms 'addiction' and 'drug habituation' have now been replaced, on the recommendation of the World Health Organization (WHO), by the term 'drug dependence'[18]. This is defined as a state, psychic and sometimes physical, resulting from the interaction of a living organism and a drug, characterized by behavioural and other responses that always include a compulsion to take the drug on a continuous or periodic basis in order to experience its psychic effects, and sometimes to avoid the discomfort of its absence. Tolerance may or may not be present. A person may be dependent on more than one drug. Thus even though an individual may initially take a drug in order to become accepted into a social group, a state may develop when he or she is obliged to continue taking the drug to avoid the withdrawal state. Drugs of dependence always produce psychological withdrawal symptoms, and some also produce physical withdrawal signs.

ALCOHOL

Ethyl alcohol is of medical importance because of the psychological, medical and social consequences of its excessive use as a beverage. Complications start to appear when more than 50 ml of alcohol is taken daily. Serious dependence usually exists when the daily intake exceeds 150–200 ml. The distinction between an alcoholic and a heavy drinker is whether the individual has control over his drinking or whether he is obliged to continue drinking excessively for psychological and physical reasons.

Alcohol is the most important drug of dependence. From consultations about alcoholism made to physicians it is calculated that 1 per cent of the population is affected. However, not all alcoholics consult their doctors and it is estimated that the incidence of alcoholism in the adult population of western Europe and North America is 5 per cent. The WHO recommend the use of the term 'alcoholism' to cover all forms of drinking problems, and instead of using the description 'alcoholic' recommend the term 'individual with an alcohol-related problem or with alcohol-dependence syndrome'. The alcohol-related problems are: psychological, medical and social.

Psychological problems

- **Chronic neural damage** Dementia; paranoia
- **Consequences of vitamin B_1 deficiency** Wernicke's encephalopathy; Korsakoff's psychosis
- **Withdrawal states** Tremor; acute confusion; delirium tremens; auditory hallucinations
- **Depression**
- **Suicide and parasuicide** are common in alcoholics, particularly when drinking has been associated with losing employment or spouse
- **Anxiety and phobias**
- **Sexual problems** Boastfulness, pseudosexuality and impotence

Medical problems

- **Neurological** Fits; peripheral neuropathy; cerebellar syndrome
- **Alimentary** Cirrhosis; alcoholic hepatitis; peptic ulcer; pancreatitis; gastritis
- **Haematological** Anaemia; bone marrow depression
- **Cardiomyopathy** Congestive cardiac failure; cardiac arrhythmias
- **Metabolic** Gout; hypoglycaemia; hypertriglyceridaemia
- **Interactions** with other drugs, particularly potentiation of other central nervous system depressants, such as hypnosedatives, antidepressants and neuroleptics

Social problems

- **Marital** and other family difficulties, including child abuse
- **Work** problems and absences
- **Accidents**, most commonly those involving driving
- **Crime** Theft, violence, road traffic offences

'At-risk' groups These are not completely definable, and why all heavy drinkers do not become dependent is not known. Nevertheless, there appears to be a familial tendency, as 25 per cent of all male relatives of alcohol-dependent individuals themselves become dependent.

Some occupations associated with a high risk of alcoholism

- Alcohol trades
- Company directors and commercial travellers
- Seamen and members of the armed forces
- Journalists and entertainers
- Doctors

The early recognition of alcoholism

The suspicion that a patient may be an alcoholic should be raised if any of the risk factors (such as familial drink problem, high-risk occupation), medical complications (such as gastritis, liver disease, late onset epilepsy), psychiatric complications (such as anxiety, depression, paranoia, attempted suicide) or social problems (such as criminal offences, marital or work difficulties) of alcohol are present. Direct questioning may produce a spuriously negative reply, but detailed structural questionnaires may be revealing. Laboratory tests may show abnormalities.

Laboratory tests which may be abnormal

- Raised aspartate and alanine aminotransferase (transaminases)
- Raised gamma-glutamyltranspeptidase
- Hypertriglyceridaemia
- Alcohol in a random blood sample
- Hyperuricaemia
- Macrocytosis
- Hypomagnesaemia
- Raised glutamate dehydrogenase
- Abnormal amino-*n*-butyric acid/leucine ratio
- Raised serum transferrin

If alcoholism is detected, it is important to assess its severity and identify aggravating and ameliorating factors.

MANAGEMENT OF ALCOHOLISM

The management of a problem drinker extends beyond the patient and his medical and psychological problems. The effects on his family and work may have to be examined and intervention may help to break the vicious circle of social malfunctioning leading to hostility and rejection, which in turn result in anxiety, depression and further escape into drink.

Controlled drinking

From an individual patient's point of view the usual aim of treatment is complete abstinence from alcohol. If this can be attained for several years, there is a striking reduction in neurotic symptoms and excellent improvement in social and economic functioning. However, if a 'cure' is possible then the patient should be able to indulge in controlled social drinking without a disastrous exacerbation of the problem. Not only would he be able to restrict his intake to (say) 2–6 units – as in 1–3 pints (1¾–5¼ litres) of bitter beer daily – but he would sip his drink slowly, be able to order alcohol, then stop drinking on his volition according to the protocol worked out with his therapist. The difficulty with allowing each patient a specific amount of alcohol is that body weight, body fat, biochemical and neurological tolerance vary in different individuals. It is not the amount but the *effect* of the alcohol which is important. Thus controlled drinking means ingestion of alcohol which is voluntarily terminated before there is any interference in intellectual, affective, physical, legal and social spheres.

Many patients who have been successfully and completely withdrawn from alcohol believe that *any* exposure to drink will produce an inevitable relapse, and controlled drinking must not be introduced in these individuals. Even if controlled drinking is a feasible aim (and this is not certain) the harm produced by a total belief in not drinking is infinitely less than that of problem drinking. The evidence in favour of controlled drinking in the treatment of alcoholism is at present inadequate. Certainly failed controlled drinkers and those with organ damage must permanently abstain from alcohol.

Social, psychiatric and occupational factors

Once a drinking problem is diagnosed, the physician must examine whether there are any social, psychiatric or occupational factors which might have increased the patient's vulnerability and which could be manipulated. At this early stage it is essential to find out how much is being drunk and the pattern of excessive consumption. Initial clinical and laboratory examination should establish the presence and severity of alcohol-associated diseases.

A patient will not stop drinking because his doctor tells him to do so, and will usually hesitate to seek medical help because of a fear of such a directive and paternalistic approach (and of its inevitable failure). To help a patient decide whether he will attempt to abstain, the doctor should not moralize, but concentrate initially in a practical manner on the social, legal and medical problems which have arisen from the drinking.

If the patient can learn to trust the doctor's attitude and feel confident that there is no question of disapproval of his behaviour, in subsequent consultations drinking behaviour can be discussed and the possible relationship between life events and drinking bouts examined. This is the most critical part of the management. During this phase it can become apparent to the patient that he has not lost control of drinking all the time, but recognizable events can start a drinking binge and other external factors can stop it.

If the patient begins to develop an interest in overcoming his drinking problems, considerable help will be needed in providing attainable targets. The enlistment of sympathetic aid from the spouse is essential; a marital therapist may provide the necessary expertise for this to work. Anxiety, depression and paranoia may also need expert treatment. It should be borne in mind that financial problems may be compounding feelings of guilt and inadequacy.

Practical therapy

The first direct approach to the drinking itself is instruction about the harmful effects of alcohol and instilling the idea that control of drinking is never completely lost. In this way the patient learns that he has control of his own future and understands the consequences of excessive drinking.

Following this stage, it is helpful if the patient keeps a record of all alcohol consumption with a note of the circumstances under which it was consumed. Drinks should be converted into units, each equivalent to 1 single tot of spirits; ½ pint (about ¼ litre) of beer; 1 glass of wine. If total abstinence is not an initial aim, then the patient must agree to stop drinking after 6 units have been consumed. The fact that stopping (and starting) drinking is under the patient's control must be stressed. Any factors which interfere with this – such as domestic arguments or heavy-drinking companions – must be identified and noted. Even when the planned programme is going wrong, the written diary of daily events must be continued. The following advice at this stage can aid the way to improvement:

- Drink with food only
- Slow down the rate of drinking
- Change drinking companion to spouse
- Change place of drinking
- Don't drink before 7.00 p.m.

Complete abstinence If complete abstinence is the aim (if controlled drinking has failed or if there are medical complications due to alcohol) then this should be attempted for three months – accompanied by a supportive programme of advice and encouragement. Tips on how to handle offers of drinks, explain abstinence, and refuse invitations to parties should be given. At the same time as individual therapy, group therapy (as with Alcoholics Anonymous) may be started. For highly motivated patients disulfiram may be a help to maintain total abstinence.

If the three-month goal has been successfully attained, then the same regime might be attempted for a longer period, say six months. However, failure during the initial three-month period should not be allowed to produce undue feelings of guilt; instead a modified programme of controlled drinking should be instituted.

Case history: life event leading to recovery

Following a divorce, a forty-five-year-old headmaster began to drink whisky during his working day. He kept his job despite being drunk during working hours, because his staff were protective and took on many of his duties. He refused any medical help.

After eighteen months he married a mathematics teacher. He has not abused alcohol since (twenty-two years ago) – and can drink socially with pleasure, without losing control or getting drunk.

Case history: suicide

A thirty-five-year-old Canadian lady with a ten-year-old son was unhappily married. She drank excessively and was frequently drunk. After a year of this behaviour she began to suffer from agitation and depression. She was prescribed amitriptyline and chlordiazepoxide. Five months later she took a half bottle of gin and approximately twenty tablets each of amitriptyline and chlordiazepoxide. She was dead on arrival at hospital.

Many alcoholics suffer from depression, and frequently commit suicide.

MANAGEMENT OF SPECIFIC ALCOHOL-RELATED SYNDROMES

Vitamin B deficiency

Wernicke's encephalopathy presents as an amnesic and confused patient who also has nystagmus, internal and external ophthalmoplegia and ataxia. Although many patients are excited, indifference and apathy may be the dominant mental state. In the Korsakoff syndrome there is loss of memory for recent events with disorientation for time and place (but not usually for person). There is a complete failure to register new memories. The patient is often relaxed, euphoric and may make up stories in order to fill in memory gaps. Both conditions are due to vitamin B_1 deficiency, although other dietary deficiencies usually coexist.

Treatment Parenteral B vitamins must be prescribed for Wernicke's encephalopathy and Korsakoff's psychosis. A suitable preparation is Parenterovite IMHP: 7 ml of the intramuscular solution (in two ampoules) contains nicotinamide 160 mg, pyridoxine hydrochloride 50 mg, riboflavine 4 mg, thiamine hydrochloride 250 mg with ascorbic acid 500 mg.

With even mild physical dependence nutritional deficiencies may develop; vitamins B_1, B_{12} and nicotinamide supplements may be required. Folic acid 15–20 mg daily is given orally if a folic acid deficiency anaemia is present.

Physical dependence

This means the appearance of clinical disorders (usually from six to eight hours) after abstinence from alcohol.

Treatment In all but the most mild cases, treatment should be carried out in hospital. Convulsions or delirium tremens may occur and continuous supervision is desirable. Alcohol should be reduced over a 14-day period.

If anxiety or tremor develop then diazepam is given on a reducing dose regime:

- 40 mg daily for 4 days
- 30 mg daily for 3 days
- 20 mg daily for 2 days
- 10 mg for 1 day

Fits are treated with intravenous diazepam or clonazepam. Chlormethiazole is also an excellent sedative, anxiolytic and anticonvulsant but it has an addiction risk. Chlorpromazine reduces panic but can precipitate fits.

Delirium tremens

Delirium tremens is a serious illness seen in heavy drinkers on withdrawal from alcohol. An infection or injury may be a precipitating factor. As little as four hours after his last drink the patient may become tense, restless and tremulous, showing extreme sensitivity to light and noise. Following this phase physical illusions and hallucinations may develop. The hallucinations, usually visual, are typically frightening and unpleasant, consisting of small animals or insects. There may also be hallucinations of touch and muscle sense, such as the feeling of floating or flying. There is insomnia, increasing restlessness and delirium. Fits may precede the delirious phase.

This illness usually lasts three to seven days and its onset may be delayed (unusually) several days after stopping alcohol. The delirium ends with a period of sleep. There is no recall of events during the illness.

Treatment The patient should be admitted to hospital immediately. Large doses of anticonvulsant anxiolytics are given (diazepam up to 100–400 mg daily). Death can occur due to circulatory failure, so plasma infusions and electrolyte correction may be required. Infections and vitamin deficiencies are also treated vigorously.

SMOKING

Tobacco smoke is a complex mixture of substances. Among these is nicotine, which is an alkaloid present in the leaves of the tobacco plant.

Nicotine has actions on the autonomic nervous system (resulting in vasoconstriction and tachycardia), carotid body (producing respiratory stimulation) and on the CNS (wakefulness, anorexia, tremor and convulsions). Nicotine is powerfully addictive. Unfortunately between one-third and one-half of smokers die as a result of smoking.

Diseases leading to illness and death from smoking

- Ischaemic heart disease
- Bronchial carcinoma
- Chronic bronchitis and emphysema
- Pulmonary heart disease
- Acute respiratory infections
- Cancers of oesophagus, lip, tongue and trachea
- Non-syphilitic aortic aneurysm
- Complications of hernia and peptic ulcer
- Peripheral vascular disease

(The incidence of Parkinson's disease and ulcerative colitis is reduced in smokers)

Giving up

As well as a powerful psychological dependence on smoking (which includes dependence on the effects of nicotine, the handling of cigarettes and the oral gratification of the procedure) there is probably a mild physical withdrawal state which includes increased appetite and constipation.

As with all drug dependence, a high degree of patient motivation is the most important factor in determining successful withdrawal. In different individuals there may be different aids to motivation. Whereas a middle-aged patient may be impressed with the possibility of premature death, this may not weigh so heavily in a younger smoker who may be more alarmed that the habit produces bad breath, stained teeth and fingernails, and unpleasant-smelling clothes. Health-conscious young adults should be told about the influence of smoking on the developing fetus and its action in accelerating the ageing of the lungs, bones and blood vessels.

Aids to stop smoking

Various aids are available to help the motivated patient stop smoking. Some people are able to stop the habit completely once they have made the decision to do so, and will weather the storms of withdrawal. It is a mistake to substitute cigar smoking, as the smoke from this will be inhaled by a cigarette addict. In those who need a more gradual withdrawal, the introduction of graded filters (which allow a decreased amount of smoke to be inhaled) can be used if the total number of cigarettes smoked is not increased. Nicotine chewing gum is now available in two strengths (2 and 4 mg). The nicotine is resin bound and although its absorption into the circulation is much slower than during smoking (and hence less satisfying), the release of nicotine is dependent on the speed of chewing the gum. Most of the nicotine is absorbed via the buccal mucosa during thirty minutes of average chewing – chewing 4 mg pieces of nicotine chewing gum every hour produces plasma nicotine levels similar to those found in heavy smokers. Nicotine chewing gum is mainly used to control withdrawal symptoms while the behavioural components of the dependence are being overcome.

Most techniques of giving up smoking give a success rate of 15–20 per cent after one year. In some series with nicotine chewing gum over 30 per cent success rates have been attained[19].

SEDATIVES

Over the last fifteen years it has become recognized that the medical use of hypnotics and anxiolytics for all but brief episodes readily produces dependence. Although the barbiturates and glutethimide, methyprylone and methaqualone can more easily produce dependence than the benzodiazepines, none of the sedatives are safe in this respect. Chloral hydrate, the antihistamines, chlormethiazole, meprobamate and ethchlorvynol can all lead to physical and psychological dependence.

Withdrawal

Withdrawal states usually consist of anxiety, insomnia, panic attacks and anorexia. Single fits or status epilepticus may develop several days after withdrawal. Delirium-tremens-like syndromes may also complicate the withdrawal picture.

Effects Patients dependent on these drugs may experience work and social problems because of sedation and impairment of judgement. Road traffic accidents are an important danger. On examination, intellectual impairment, poor brain–eye–hand coordination and shortened attention span may be recognized. Nystagmus, ataxia and other evidence of the cerebellar syndrome can develop.

Treatment Although many aspects of the withdrawal state respond to the neuroleptic drugs, these agents (such as chlorpromazine) should not be used, because they may precipitate fits. The benzodiazepines are more suitable. If status epilepticus occurs, intravenous diazepam (usually 5–20 mg) or clonazepam (0.5–2 mg) may be effective. Failing a response to intravenous benzodiazepines, intravenous thiopentone sodium with a muscle relaxant will be required.

STIMULANTS

The stimulant drugs of abuse include the amphetamine group and cocaine. Although they do not produce a physical withdrawal state, psychological dependence may be severe.

Amphetamines and cocaine

These drugs are used for their own euphoriant effects and also in order to antagonize the sedative and sexual inhibitory effects of the barbiturates and narcotics. The amphetamines ('speed') can produce hypertensive reactions, agitation and paranoid schizophrenia-like states with hallucinations.

Cocaine ('snow', 'coke') can produce a similar or more intense stimulatory and euphoric action to the amphetamines. A toxic psychosis can develop with delusions of grandeur and of strength. Fits and hypertension can also result, and death can be caused by cardiac arrhythmias.

The amphetamines are taken orally or by injection. Cocaine is degraded in the stomach but is well absorbed from the buccal or nasal mucosa. The intense vasoconstriction produced by cocaine can result in mucosal gangrene and perforation of the nasal septum. Cocaine is also injected intravenously.

HALLUCINOGENS

All the stimulants, anticholinergics and some other drugs can produce hallucinations. The hallucinogenic drugs include those listed in the table opposite.

SOLVENT ABUSE (SNIFFING)

The growing problem of solvent sniffing is frequently a group activity. The volatile substance is inhaled from a plastic bag or an impregnated cloth. The results of inhaling any of a wide range of organic solvents are the acute mental and physical changes usually associated with alcohol. Once the habit has become established, the subject may go on to alcohol abuse.

Hallucinogenic drugs

Stimulants

- Methylphenidate, phenmetrazine and phencyclidine ('angel dust')
- Cocaine
- Amphetamine derivatives
  - Amphetamine
  - Dextroamphetamine
  - Methamphetamine
  - Dimethoxyamphetamine (methoxymethylamphetamine; STP; DOM)
  - 4, 3-methylenedioxyamphetamine (MDA)

Anticholinergics

- Atropine, hyoscine and stramonium
- Benztropine and benzhexol
- Angel trumpets

Cannabis preparations

Derivatives of 5-HT

- Mescaline: from peyote cactus
- Psilocybin and psilocin: from psilocybe and stropharia mushrooms
- D-lysergic acid diethylamide (LSD): from ergot
- Dimethyltryptamine (DMT)
- Harmaline

Solvents

Amyl nitrite

The volatile substances which are constituents of glues, cleaning fluids and petrol include toluene, benzene, acetone, *n*-hexane, trichloroethylene, carbon tetrachloride, methylene chloride and butane.

The chronic effects of sniffing vary according to the chemical used, but lability of mood, fatigue and anorexia are common. Benzene can produce bone marrow depression and cerebral atrophy. A peripheral neuropathy may result from *n*-hexane. Hepatic and renal damage can be produced by toluene and xylene.

NARCOTIC ANALGESICS (OPIOIDS)

These agents include several minor analgesics such as codeine, dihydrocodeine and dextropropoxyphene, and major analgesics such as pethidine, methadone, morphine and diamorphine (heroin).

The narcotic analgesics are effective by mouth but those who abuse these drugs frequently self-administer them by intravenous or subcutaneous injection, or by sniffing or inhalation of the volatalized substance to experience anxiolytic actions and relief from withdrawal symptoms rapidly and intensely (called 'buzz'). In a normal individual morphine produces unpleasant sensations such as sedation, giddiness, feelings of faintness, and vomiting. However, in a patient experiencing pain or in an addict suffering from the withdrawal syndrome, the administration of narcotic analgesics produces euphoria.

Dependence on these drugs is both physical and psychological, and even the weakest analgesics in this series can be addictive. Nevertheless the severity of the withdrawal state varies roughly with the analgesic potency of the drug. There are, however, important exceptions to this – particularly those analgesics (such as pentazocine) which have mixed agonist and antagonist activity. Such drugs produce less anxiolytic and euphoric action compared with pure agonists, and can even produce dysphoric states, which may consist of feelings of uneasiness or panic accompanied by unpleasant hallucinations.

The narcotic addict profile

The number of narcotic addicts is continuing to rise in Britain. At the present time the majority of dependent individuals did not originally come in contact with these drugs in a medical and therapeutic context. In other words, the epidemic addict has voluntarily induced the state in himself. There is no such thing as an addiction-prone personality. It appears that prolonged and repeated exposure is necessary in order to become dependent. The young are possibly more vulnerable to peer pressures to conform with group activity. Other pleasure-seeking behaviour is often present within drug-abusing groups, such as early experience of smoking, alcohol and sex. There may be a history of truancy, poor work record and a record of criminal behaviour.

Acute illnesses caused by opiate abuse

Respiratory depression and liver damage Although tolerance to the euphoric effects of the narcotic analgesics may be considerable, there is much less tolerance to their respiratory depressant actions. Even relatively weak analgesics such as dextropropoxyphene can, in large doses, lead to fatal respiratory depression. Dextropropoxyphene is readily available in Britain in the form of Distalgesic tablets, in which it is mixed with paracetamol. Excessive amounts of Distalgesic not only produce respiratory depression, but can lead to fatal liver failure due to the paracetamol.

Infections Up to 8 per cent of opiate addicts are found to have infective endocarditis when admitted to hospital. Viral hepatitis and chronic active hepatitis are common and are presumably due to poor injection technique and venereal infection. There can be osteomyelitis and skin infections, and venereal diseases are very common.

Organ damage This may follow anoxic episodes, adulterants in the drugs, emboli and immunological disease. The syndromes encountered include glomerulonephritis, transverse myelitis, postanoxic brain damage, retinal and limb embolization, and pulmonary hypertension.

Cardiac arrhythmias These include supraventricular tachyarrhythmias, heart block, ventricular ectopic beats.

Respiratory system These include aspiration pneumonia, bronchiectasis, pulmonary oedema, lung abscess and ventilation-perfusion defects.

Acquired immune-deficiency syndrome (AIDS) The symptoms here are proneness to overwhelming infections and tumours.

Gastrointestinal These include severe constipation and intestinal obstruction.

Acute overdose This may present either as pulmonary oedema or as a severe hypoxic episode (complicated by cardiac arrhythmias in 25 per cent of patients).

Obstetric problems The addict mother does not often attend an antenatal clinic. The newborn infant usually has a low birthweight and may be born before term; within four days of delivery, a withdrawal state may begin, consisting of irritability, tremors, vomiting, diarrhoea, sneezing, yawning, respiratory difficulties and (uncommonly) fits. The condition may be controlled with chlorpromazine, but if fits develop diazepam is used.

Treatment of dependence

The ideal aim of treatment is complete and permanent withdrawal from opiates, but this is not often attained unless the patient is motivated to reach this goal. The only alternative is to supply the addict with his opiate (or methadone as an alternative opiate) in such a way that he cannot sell or give away the drug. As heroin or other major narcotic is gradually withdrawn oral methadone is introduced in its place. When the patient is stabilized at 100 mg (or less) daily, he may suffer no major toxic effects from this and yet be free from physical withdrawal symptoms and from psychological craving for more dangerous opiates. Opiate antagonists (such as naloxone) and partial agonists (such as pentazocine) are contraindicated, and can produce a withdrawal state.

Withdrawal The withdrawal state usually starts 8 hours after the last dose of opiate and reaches a peak at 36–72 hours. The peak is early with the more severely addicting drugs (morphine, diamorphine and pethidine) but occurs later and is less severe with methadone. At first the patient becomes sleepy, unhappy, cries and experiences rhinorrhoea and sweating. He may fall asleep but at about 24 hours after the last dose wakes and suffers chills, excessive sweating, gooseflesh, nausea, vomiting, diarrhoea and severe abdominal cramps. The blood pressure is labile and can be considerably raised and accompanied by alterations in heart rate. Cardiac arrhythmias and pulmonary oedema may also develop. The withdrawal state is not usually fatal but sleep disturbances, nightmares and craving for the drug may last for many months. For patients who can be withdrawn from the narcotic without methadone replacement, diazepam is effective in controlling these late withdrawal effects.

CANNABIS

Cannabis consists of a mixture of substances in the resin of the flowering tops (hashish) or from the chopped leaves and stalks (marihuana) of *Cannabis sativa*. The active constituents are highly lipid soluble and include delta(δ)-9 tetrahydrocannabinol (THC). The main active metabolite of THC is the 1-hydroxy derivative.

Psychological effects

These vary according to dose, route of administration and social setting of the administration. Smoking a cigarette containing up to 5 mg of THC produces feelings of relaxation, sleepiness and euphoria. Driving ability is impaired, and learning ability and short-term memory are inhibited. These effects are similar to those of alcohol. However, in addition, goal-directed behaviour is suppressed, there is early disturbance of balance, reduction in muscular strength and often some elements of a confusional state are present – in particular a disturbance in time sense, with confusion of past, present and future.

Experienced smokers may feel a more keen perception of auditory and visual stimuli, and perception of sounds and colours may take on an altered quality. High doses can produce hallucinations as a component of a paranoid psychosis or a frank acute confusional state. Perception of time, sounds and vision may become very disturbed. Panic attacks are usually terrifying ('bad trip') and may recur in attacks after habitual use of the drug has ceased ('flashbacks').

Physical effects

These include conjunctival injection, bronchitis, pharyngitis and tachycardia. Chronic smokers can develop bronchitis and airways obstruction, apathy and reduction in drive and ambition.

LONG-TERM RESULTS IN TREATMENT OF DRUG DEPENDENCE

The long-term results in the treatment of drug abuse are poor in many series[20]. However, 'experimental' illicit drug-taking is probably common and is not usually followed by dependence.

In severe alcoholism, treatment results in long-term abstinence in only 15–20 per cent of subjects.

PRACTICAL POINTS

- The aims of treating dependence to alcohol and other drugs are withdrawal, and restoration of normal social functioning.
- The first step in treatment of alcoholism is for the patient to admit that there is a problem. Constant support and encouragement are essential and the use of group therapy (as in Alcoholics Anonymous) may be beneficial.
- In alcoholism limited goals – such as restricting daily intake to an agreed amount for six weeks – should be agreed on by patient and physician.
- Alteration in associated behaviour – such as only taking alcohol with food and drinking slowly can be aimed at. How to avoid solitary drinking and avoiding company which encourages alcohol abuse may be discussed with the patient and spouse.
- Once the initial goal has been attained then further targets can be set (e.g. complete abstinence for three months); failure must not be followed by any suggestion of rejection. Long-term aims may have to be modified from complete abstinence to limited, controlled and supervised drug/alcohol use.
- Associated mental illness (e.g. depression) and social problems (e.g. unemployment, marital crisis) have to be tackled at the same time as reduction in drug intake.
- In smoking, a high degree of patient motivation is important, and there are various aids available, such as graded filters or nicotine chewing gum.
- Neuroleptic drugs should not be used in the treatment of sedative and alcohol withdrawal, because they may precipitate fits.

8
Placebos and their actions

BACKGROUND

The use of pharmacologically inactive substances by physicians is an emotive subject. There are overtones of dishonesty and quackery, as it is widely thought that placebos are without significant effect. Furthermore, there are fears that if a patient who had experienced a change in the symptoms of his disease after taking a placebo discovered the nature of his treatment he would suffer loss of face. Many physicians do not administer placebos (as such) because of the unethical overtones of such a practice. Perhaps the most important aspect of the study of the placebo response is that any type of treatment can produce effects which cannot be attributed to the physiological actions of the treatment. Factors which are not part of the specific treatment may be of great importance in determining the outcome of therapy. Because of this it has been suggested that a distinction be made between drug response (the effects produced following administration of a drug) and drug effect (the effects which are attributable to the pharmacological actions of the drug).

EFFECTS OF PLACEBOS

Placebos can have positive effects when a symptom or disease reacts favourably, but they can also have negative effects which produce worsening of the patient's condition or result in toxic effects.

Because of the considerable activity of placebos, it is necessary to carry out many drug trials on a double-blind basis – neither patient nor physician knowing which treatment is being used. Single-blind methods – in which only the patient does not know which treatment is being given – are not always so satisfactory, because the patient is profoundly influenced by the expectations of the therapist, and by his view of the trial.

Placebos can have effects which have in the past been thought to be the properties only of pharmacologically active substances.

Placebo effects

- Toxic effects
- Time/effect relationship
- Cumulation
- Hangover
- Weakening of therapeutic effect as the symptoms become more severe

Placebo composition

The physical form of the placebo can modify its effect. Colourless or tasteless medications are considered inferior to coloured and bitter-tasting ones. Some observers have found red and white capsules produce more toxicity than green and yellow capsules. However, identical iron preparations cause more gastrointestinal disturbances when coloured green than when they are yellow or red. There has been a suggestion that laxatives should be brown and taste salty, while hypnotics should be bitter. Many patients feel that large tablets or capsules are particularly potent. Multicoloured spherules within a transparent capsule may also suggest particular power of action.

There are conflicting results as to whether injections are more effective than oral therapy; but if a placebo injection is given for pain, then injection into the painful site is more analgesic than if given elsewhere[21, 22, 23].

CIRCUMSTANCES OF ADMINISTERING PLACEBOS

Placebos are extensively used in drug testing on normal volunteers and in clinical trials. Apart from this type of situation, doctors do not often give placebos to patients for therapeutic reasons; although, unfortunately, some doctors and nurses do administer them as a semi-punitive measure. A survey of two university hospitals in New Mexico revealed that medical staff (erroneously) prescribed placebos to patients to indicate that 'pain was not real'[24]. They tended to be given to unpopular patients to relieve feelings of aggression in the medical staff and to label these patients as undeserving of 'real drugs'. Happily, this is an uncommon practice.

Drugs with placebo-like actions

More usually, active agents are used which, without the physician's knowledge, have an effect on the symptom or disease that does not differ from placebo.

Meprobamate The use of the anxiolytic and hypnotic meprobamate is a case in point. This became very popular, and was widely and successfully used in the treatment of anxiety states and insomnia. After many years of use, double-blind trials showed it was no more effective than placebo in the doses usually prescribed[24].

Anticholinergic drugs and other agents Anticholinergic drugs with weak ganglion-blocking activity, such as propantheline and poldine, have been used to treat pain due to peptic ulcer. In large doses they decrease the result of the vagal drive to the secretion of pepsin and acid in the stomach, and they also reduce smooth muscle spasm. They exert no pharmacological action in the doses used.

In a similar way patients may experience relief of symptoms from vitamins, plant extracts, mineral supplements and animal products without any pharmacological basis for this.

Non-drug therapy

Non-drug forms of therapy can also exert powerful placebo effects. Certainly operations and other procedures, such as ECT, involving general anaesthesia carry a powerful healing effect from the incidental aspects of the procedures alone. Some operations which in the past had produced good results have been demonstrated to have identical efficacy to placebos. These include gastrojejunostomy for peptic ulcer, sympathectomy for hypertension, ligation and transplantation of the internal mammary artery for angina, and probably the majority of tonsillectomies and adenoidectomies[24].

PAIN

The sensation of pain is a complex experience. Apart from the primitive appreciation of the quality and intensity of the experience, accompanying emotional responses not only colour the sensation of pain but can also affect the threshold at which pain is appreciated. Past experience of pain, depression and anxiety all act to increase the suffering, distress and intensity of the experience. Pain itself is hyperalgesic, and effective medical relief of pain lowers the threshold and diminishes the suffering from subsequent painful episodes. Loneliness also has an adverse effect, while company, particularly of interested, sympathetic and understanding people, can alone provide relief. Past experience and future expectations are important. In chronic terminal illness much suffering is caused because pain under these circumstances tends to be chronic, has no purpose and may well become more severe. By contrast, soldiers wounded in battle appear to demand morphine less often than postoperative civilian patients in hospital with similar somatic trauma. This has been attributed to the relief and thankfulness the soldiers must feel on being removed from the battlefield, finding themselves alive and with the prospect of recovery[25].

Pain and reaction to placebos

In clinical conditions such as angina pectoris and postoperative pain placebos produce a significant reduction in pain in about one-third of patients.

Angina pectoris is particularly prone to placebo responses. The pattern exhibited underlines the importance of the expectations of the physician and patient. In a review of 1187 patients in 13 studies which tested 5 different inactive treatments, Herbert Benson and David McCallie found that the pattern was consistent; initial trials by enthusiasts produced 70–90 per cent effectiveness[26]. This decreased to 30–40 per cent in later trials which were presumably carried out by more sceptical investigators. The authors quote Trousseau, the nineteenth-century French physician who wrote: 'You should treat as many patients as possible with the new drugs while they still have the power to heal.'

There do not appear to be two distinct types of individual – for example, placebo reactors and placebo non-reactors – all treatments and all patients produce and respond to non-specific effects respectively. The responders are not particularly suggestible or neurotic. However, spontaneous changes in the disease and differences in the setting of the pain can greatly alter the intensity of symptoms.

Compared with non-steroidal anti-inflammatory agents (NSAIDs) and with narcotic analgesics, some trials have showed that the efficacy of placebos is about 50 per cent that of the active drug when measured on a scale of pain severity[24]. However, active drugs may raise the pain threshold while placebos do not generally do this.

Anxiety One important determinant of pain relief by placebos is the presence of concomitant anxiety. It has to be present initially and then reduced by the circumstances of the therapy. If anxiety is absent or if the clinical situation is such that anxiety is maintained at a high level, then the placebo (and much other treatment) will not be effective. This observation probably explains why placebos are relatively ineffective in experimentally produced pain[24]. Here only 3 per cent of subjects respond. In these the pain relief is, on an average, about 15 per cent. In the laboratory, the subjects have little or no anxiety about the procedure, they trust the skill and humanity of the experimenters and, perhaps most important of all, know that they can stop the pain at any moment.

TOXIC EFFECTS OF PLACEBOS

One of the benefits of including a placebo in a double-blind trial of a new drug is as a baseline for toxicity. Placebo administration can cause a wide range of toxic actions.

Toxic actions caused by placebos

- Anorexia
- Dyspepsia
- Constipation
- Diarrhoea
- Headache
- Paraesthesiae
- Rashes
- Sleepiness
- Sleeplessness
- Tremulousness
- Dizziness
- Palpitations

Sometimes sudden collapse can be provoked by placebo – superficially similar to anaphylactic shock. These patients may become pale and sweat before fainting. The blood pressure can fall during this reaction, and even angioneurotic oedema of the lips and generalized urticaria can follow.

Addiction to placebos can also occur. This is an uncommon problem, but when it develops in a person who had previously been dependent on a more dangerous drug it can be considered a great benefit.

MECHANISMS OF PLACEBOS

The personalities of the medical attendants, and the relationship between them and the patient have been mentioned earlier in this chapter. One influence of this interaction can be a reduction in anxiety – which in itself may alter the perception of some symptoms (such as pain) and can alter disease mechanisms (such as gastric secretion, gut motility and bronchial reactivity).

Some of the reaction to placebos may well be triggered by spontaneous fluctuations in the course of the disease, but once a trend has been experienced, psychological factors can maintain it by powerful effects on physiological function. For example, the discussion of an emotionally laden and anger-provoking topic can produce hyperaemia of the gastric mucosa and increases in acid and pepsin secretion beyond that which can be produced by standard doses of histamine. Placebos may produce vomiting with all the concomitant changes in alimentary activity: cessation of gastric and oesphageal peristalsis, closure of the pylorus, salivation, lachrimation and nasal secretion. Conversely, when placebos abolish nausea they can cause the sudden appearance of gastric motility and opening of the pylorus.

Cerebral factors can cause sweating, localized vasodilatation, tachycardia, urticaria and even changes in the eosinophil count and plasma lipoproteins.

Positive conditioning, as by a past history of successful therapy by the physician, can sustain and amplify the placebo response.

Problems which have arisen because of psychological factors are probably the most amenable to dramatic cures mediated by placebos. These include pain due to muscle tension, loss of appetite, decrease in libido, insomnia and minor skin blemishes.

PRACTICAL POINTS

- A distinction should be made between drug response and drug effect.
- Placebos can have positive effects when a symptom or disease reacts favourably, but their negative effects can produce worsening of the patient's condition or result in toxic effects.
- Non-drug therapy can also have powerful placebo effects.
- In clinical conditions such as angina pectoris and postoperative pain, placebos significantly reduce pain in about a third of patients.
- Placebos can produce various toxic actions, and can also cause addiction.
- Placebos are probably most successful in the treatment of pain caused by muscular tension; loss of appetite; decrease in libido; insomnia; and minor skin blemishes.

9
Drug-induced problems

Conditions that can be induced by drugs cover a wide spectrum. In this chapter we deal with six areas: sexual dysfunction in male and female, depression, nightmares, psychoses, anxiety, and delirium.

SEXUAL DYSFUNCTION IN THE MALE

Normal male sexual activity depends on cerebral and genital factors, both of which can be influenced by hormonal and neural changes. The physiological process is complex and incompletely understood. For example, androgens not only govern the maintenance of secondary sexual characteristics in the male but heighten libido (in males and females), presumably by an action on specific receptors in cerebral neurones. It is also possible that hormones may facilitate erection. Apart from the possibility that androgens may have such an action, it has been postulated that an intestinal hormone, vasoactive intestinal peptide (VIP), may be an erection-promoting hormone.

Local neural control of erection is via the pelvic parasympathetic outflow (sacral segments 2 and 3) which is cholinergic and muscarinic. This outflow is activated by a reflex initiated by touch receptors in the genital skin and also by cerebral stimuli. A contribution to erection is also made by sympathetic vasodilator (β_2) nerves and possibly by circulating adrenaline.

Ejaculation is preceded by contraction of internal sphincter to prevent retrograde discharge of semen into the bladder. Ejaculation is mediated via sympathetic nerves (causing contraction of the seminal vesicles, vas deferens and the internal sphincter), and by activity of somatic efferent nerves which cause contraction of the bulbar muscles.

Although a wide range of drugs can reduce or abolish sexual activity in the male, psychological factors are a more common cause of sexual dysfunction.

Drugs which have this type of action may act on sexual arousal or on peripheral mechanisms.

Sexual arousal

Testosterone is required for sexual arousal and its deficiency usually results in impotence. Oestrogens (such as stilboestrol), hydroxyprogesterone caproate and cyproterone have antiandrogenic activity, decrease libido and can produce impotence.

Drugs increasing or decreasing sexual arousal Sedatives, such as the benzodiazepines and alcohol, may reduce arousal but can sometimes facilitate sexual activity by their anxiolytic action. The neuroleptics such as chlorpromazine and thioridazine reduce libido by a general sedative action, and also by a reduction in autonomic outflow and by induced depression. The action of the neuroleptics in this respect is complex and several of their peripheral actions also lead to sexual difficulties.

Administration of spironolactone and cimetidine can occasionally be associated with erectile failure. The mechanisms involved are not known, but there is evidence that this is due to a central action, possibly by interference with sexually arousing properties of endogenous testosterone.

The narcotic analgesics decrease sexual desire. Diamorphine addicts are frequently impotent or have reduced sexual activity.

Drugs which can produce depression, such as methyldopa, clonidine, fenfluramine and antihistamines (H_1) may, by this mechanism, reduce libido.

Drugs affecting male sexual arousal

- Benzodiazepines
- Alcohol
- Neuroleptics
- Spironolactone
- Cimetidine
- Narcotic analgesics
- Methyldopa
- Clonidine
- Fenfluramine
- Antihistamines

Peripheral mechanisms

Anticholinergic drugs These can lead to erectile failure because of a block of parasympathetically mediated engorgement and vasodilatation in the penis. In this way impotence can result from some of the neuroleptics, tricyclic antidepressants, monoamine oxidase inhibitors, anticholinergic antiparkinsonian drugs (such as benzhexol and benztropine), H_1 antihistamines, disopyramide, hyoscine, atropine and atropine analogues used as antiasthma agents.

Sympathomimetic drugs Drugs such as ephedrine and amphetamine can also interfere with erection and produce premature ejaculation.

Antisympathetic drugs These can produce both impotence and failure of ejaculation. Both these conditions are common with the antihypertensive adrenergic neurone blockers bethanidine and guanethidine. Impotence or ejaculatory failure can occur with methyldopa. Beta-blocking drugs rarely produce erectile failure but do not otherwise interfere with ejaculation, presumably because of blockade of β_2 vasodilatory fibre activity in the cavernous vasculature in the penis.

By contrast, the contraction of the smooth muscle of the seminal vesicles and of the vas deferens at the beginning of ejaculation is innervated by alpha-sympathetic fibres. These actions are not affected by beta-blockers but they may be prevented by alpha-blockers such as phenoxybenzamine and indoramin, both of which can produce failure of ejaculation. Surprisingly, prazosin shows this toxic effect more rarely than indoramin.

Some of the neuroleptic drugs have alpha-adrenoceptor peripheral effects and can cause ejaculatory failure or retrograde ejaculation. Thioridazine commonly has this action, but the piperazine phenothiazines and haloperidol do not.

Vasodilator drugs These do not usually lead to sexual difficulties. Hydralazine, for example, has rarely been reported to cause impotence.

The administration of thiazide and other benzothiadiazine diuretics is frequently associated with impotence. The mechanism is unknown, but the incidence of impotence is high in hypertensive patients and they may be particularly sensitive to the vasodilatory effects of these diuretics. Also the depletion of salt from cells produced by diuretics appears to reduce vascular reactivity.

Case history: impotence with diuretics

> Mr J., the owner of a sports shop, aged forty-two, was found to be mildly hypertensive on a routine medical examination for an insurance policy. He was sent to a hypertension clinic, where bendrofluazide 5 mg once a day was prescribed. His standing blood pressure fell on this regime from 158/102 to 140/94 over the course of three weeks. However, on his follow-up visit, direct questioning revealed that he had become impotent since starting the diuretic. His drug regime was changed to labetalol 100 mg three times a day. In four weeks his standing blood pressure was 132/88 and his potency had returned.

Potentiation of sexual activity in the male

Parkinson's disease In some patients with this condition the administration of levodopa causes an increase in sexual activity. This could possibly be due to a primary action of dopamine on libido – but other factors, such as improved mobility and reduction of depression, may also be operating.

Hypogonadal males frequently experience an increase in libido when given testosterone – but with normal males the effect on libido is unpredictable and a fall in sperm count can also result.

Impotent, infertile males with hyperprolactinaemia may have the condition reversed with bromocriptine.

Homosexuals frequently use nitrites or nitrates to potentiate orgasm, but other actions such as relaxation of the anal sphincter may encourage their use in this group. It is possible that abuse of nitrites leads to immunosuppression and possibly contribute to AIDS (see page 101).

Aphrodisiacs No agent is known which has aphrodisiac properties. Alcohol, other sedatives, harmaline and cannabis derivatives have a reputation for increasing libido – but what action they may have is probably due to anxiolytic effects. The placebo response in this field is considerable and makes accurate study very difficult.

DRUGS AND LIBIDO IN THE FEMALE

Libido is regularly reduced in the female by drugs which produce depression such as methyldopa and clonidine. Sedatives have an unpredictable effect, but in some people alcohol and other central nervous system depressants increase libido.

Females who abuse cannabis, cocaine and amphetamine sometimes claim either an increase in libido or potentiation of orgasm by these substances.

The effect of the oral combined contraceptive varies in different women. Libido may be increased or decreased. These actions may be complex. Those whose sexual activity was previously inhibited by a fear of pregnancy may enjoy greater relaxation while on the pill. Women who experience a mid-cycle peak of libido may find that the pill abolishes this. Those who experienced no such cyclical change without the pill may develop a late cycle peak, possibly partly associated with a reduction in premenstrual tension. As in the male, no true aphrodisiac is known for the female.

Drugs affecting female libido

- Methyldopa
- Clonidine
- Alcohol
- Central nervous system depressants
- Oral combined contraceptives
- Cannabis, cocaine and amphetamines (claimed)

DRUG-INDUCED DEPRESSION

Drowsiness and sedation produced by drugs are not themselves depressive reactions. However, many therapeutic agents can induce changes of mood identical to psychotic depression, such as loss of interest and enthusiasm, physical and mental slowing, thoughts of unworthiness and suicide, hypochondriasis and tearfulness. Successful suicide can result. A large number of types of drug can produce depression, and some may be classified as follows.

Antihypertensive agents

Many untreated hypertensives feel perfectly well (possibly even better than non-hypertensive individuals). When they start treatment they usually feel weak, dizzy and lacking in energy. In addition some of the hypotensive agents can produce depression. Reserpine is not now used in Britain as a standard treatment for hypertension because serious depressive illness appears in 10–20 per cent of patients treated in this way. Methyldopa usually produces sedation and depression sometimes develops. Clonidine produces similar effects.

Beta-adrenoceptor blockers do not usually cause depression, but those which penetrate into the brain (such as propranolol and oxprenolol) can cause nightmares and are (rarely) associated with depression.

Hormones

Drug-induced problems In the 1976 Boston Collaborative Drug Surveillance Program it was found that prednisolone was the most common cause of drug-induced serious psychiatric illness in hospital wards. Glucocorticoids in general and adrenocorticotrophic hormone (ACTH) can cause a range of psychotic reactions including mania, hypomania and depression. The latter is the most common psychological disturbance due to steroids.

The contraceptive pill Mood changes frequently occur during the menstrual cycle – particularly in premenstrual lowering of mood. The oral contraceptives are associated with depression in 4–6 per cent of women, which is a higher incidence than in a control series. Once depression has occurred it is likely to recur even with a different pill. Both oestrogen and progestogen may contribute to the depression, but depression associated with the pill is usually mild, so tricyclic antidepressants are not often required. Although experts in mental illness can find no evidence of pyridoxine deficiency in contraceptive-induced depression, patients and doctors in family planning clinics say that pyridoxine may help this complication.

Neuroleptics

Depression and suicide have occurred in patients with schizophrenia or hypomania treated with neuroleptics (see Chapter 2). Both of these diseases when untreated can lead to suicide, but the incidence of depression is higher when neuroleptics are used. The drugs most frequently associated with suicidal depression are chlorpromazine, thioridazine and depot injections of fluphenazine and flupenthixol.

Drug withdrawal

Abusers of cocaine, amphetamines, phenmetrazine and other stimulants characteristically experience hypersomnia and depression on withdrawal (see Chapter 7). Strangely, fenfluramine, which itself can produce depression during treatment, can also cause depression if it is rapidly withdrawn.

Analgesics

The narcotic analgesics are usually sedating (see Chapter 7). The partial opiate agonists, such as pentazocine, can produce dysphoria and depression.

The anti-inflammatory analgesic indomethacin causes central nervous system changes in about 10 per cent of users, including headache, confusion, hallucinations and depression.

Levodopa

Drugs which cause stimulation of dopamine receptors – in particular levodopa and bromocriptine – often cause elation in patients with Parkinson's disease, but can produce depression instead.

Hypnosedatives

Hypnotics and anxiolytics can lead to a lowering of the spirits and depressive illness may develop (see Chapter 6). The benzodiazepines have in this way led to suicide. Alcohol abusers may suffer a wide range of mental illnesses including depression.

VIVID DREAMS AND NIGHTMARES

These can be caused by some of the hypotensive drugs, in particular the beta-blockers which penetrate the central nervous system. Other hypotensives associated with vivid dreams are methyldopa, clonidine and reserpine.

The antispasticity drug, baclofen, can also increase dreaming. Fenfluramine is a potent cause of nightmares. Antiparkinsonian drugs, in particular amantadine, may also produce nightmares.

Withdrawal of alcohol, hypnotics and anxiolytics all cause sleep disturbances with frequent wakening due to vivid dreams (see Chapters 6 and 7).

Drugs causing vivid dreams and nightmares

- Beta-blockers
- Methyldopa
- Clonidine
- Reserpine
- Baclofen
- Antiparkinsonian drugs
- Alcohol, hypnotic and anxiolytic withdrawal

DRUG-INDUCED PSYCHOSES

Synthetic and naturally occurring glucocorticoids and corticotrophin can induce schizophrenic-like states as well as affective disorders. Less commonly, schizoaffective psychoses occur in women at the beginning of oral contraceptive use.

Psychotic reactions can result from a wide range of anticholinergic agents, including the atropine-like drugs used in the treatment of Parkinson's disease (such as benztropine) and bronchitis (such as ipratropium). Scopolamine, which is used as a premedication drug, can produce unpredictable violent outbursts.

The sympathomimetic central stimulants such as amphetamine, phentermine and diethylpropion may induce schizophrenic-like hallucinations and paranoia. Cocaine has very similar actions to these drugs.

Psychotic reactions and hallucinations may, rarely, be provoked by phenytoin, carbamazepine, isoniazid, disulfiram and metronidazole. In the elderly such mental changes can result from administration of cardiac glycosides.

A number of drugs of abuse can cause hallucinations, including LSD, stimulants, cannabis, mescaline, psilocybin in mushrooms, phencyclidine (angel dust) and a variety of organic solvents (see Chapter 7).

Drugs which cause stimulation of central dopamine receptors such as levodopa, bromocriptine and amantadine can all induce schizophrenic-like hallucinations.

Drugs causing psychoses

- Glucocorticoids
- Corticotrophin
- Oral contraceptives
- Many anticholinergic agents
- Sympathomimetic central stimulants
- Phenytoin
- Carbamazepine
- Isoniazid
- Disulfiram
- Metronidazole
- Cardiac glycosides
- Hallucinogenics
- Central dopamine receptor stimulants
- Amantadine

DRUG-INDUCED ANXIETY

Sympathomimetic amines such as adrenaline, ephedrine and amphetamine can produce feelings of apprehension, anxiety and panic. In addition, drugs which have mainly

Drugs causing anxiety

- Sympathomimetic amines
- Drugs with mainly peripheral sympathetic actions
- Hypoglycaemics
- Thyroid hormones
- Stimulatory antidepressants
- Stimulatory anticholinergics
- Hypnotic and alcohol withdrawal

peripheral sympathetic actions (such as tremor and palpitations) can secondarily lead to genuine feelings of fear.

Hypoglycaemic agents such as insulin and sulphonylureas can cause anxiety due to sympathetic activation as a consequence of a fall in blood glucose. Similarly, overtreatment of hypothyroidism with thyroid hormones can produce tremulousness and nervousness.

Some of the stimulatory antidepressants such as imipramine, protriptyline, MAOIs and nomifensine may cause feelings of agitation. Atropine and other stimulatory anticholinergics can also precipitate anxiety.

Severe panic can result from withdrawal of benzodiazepines, barbiturates and other hypnotics and alcohol.

DRUG-INDUCED DELIRIUM

In the elderly an acute confusional state (delirium) can readily be induced by anxiolytics and hypnotics – particularly barbiturates, glutethimide and meprobamate, but benzodiazepines, chloral hydrate and chlormethiazole can have the same effect.

Drugs causing delirium in the elderly

- Anxiolytics
- Hypnotics
- Anticholinergic antiparkinsonian drugs
- Cardiac glycosides
- Hypotensives
- Diuretics
- Cimetidine
- Phenytoin
- Chloroquine
- Isoniazid
- Levodopa
- Amantadine

The elderly can also experience acute confusion following treatment with anticholinergic antiparkinsonian drugs, cardiac glycosides, hypotensive agents and diuretics. Less commonly delirium is caused by cimetidine, phenytoin, chloroquine, isoniazid, levodopa and amantadine. (See also Chapter 5.)

Case history: drug-induced confusion

A retired orthopaedic surgeon aged seventy-four had suffered from increasing difficulty in sleeping, wandering about the house at night for three months. One morning he was found by his wife lying in the hall of their house. He could not stand, was confused and his speech was very indistinct. He improved over the course of the day, but a neurologist was called, as a stroke was suspected. In his history the neurologist discovered that the surgeon frequently took a double whisky and Sodium Amytal (both self-prescribed) together with chlormethiazole (prescribed by his family physician). When all sedation was stopped, the sleep difficulties resolved.

The original fall and confusion were attributed to effects of sedatives in a patient suffering from cerebral ischaemia.

PRACTICAL POINTS

- Drugs which can produce depression, such as methyldopa, clonidine, fenfluramine and antihistamines, can reduce libido in both males and females.
- Prednisolone appears to be the most common cause of drug-induced serious psychiatric illness.
- Synthetic and naturally occurring glucocorticoids and corticotrophin can induce schizophrenic-like states and affective disorders.
- Suicidal depression is associated with neuroleptics such as chlorpromazine, thioridazine, and depot injections of fluphenazine and flupenthixol.
- Certain sympathomimetic amines can cause anxiety feelings.
- Delirium can be caused in the elderly by anxiolytics and hypnotics.

10
Anomalies of eating

Two common anomalies of eating are eating too much and too little. Obesity and anorexia nervosa are dealt with in this chapter.

OBESITY

About 20 per cent of adults in western Europe and North America are obese. Only rarely is this due to a recognized treatable biochemical–endocrinological–neural disorder. In the majority no underlying disease can be found, although the condition is often familial.

Obesity is associated with risks to health in proportion to the degree of overweight. The risks are not apparent until the weight is more than 10 per cent above the ideal for the subject's height and build. The medical problems associated with bodyweights over twice the ideal are such that lifespan is greatly curtailed. Many of the risks are not inevitable consequences of obesity, but are significantly associated with it – diabetes mellitus, hyperlipoproteinaemia with consequent atherosclerotic disease, and hypertension. Gross obesity causes mechanical impairment of diaphragmatic movement and blood flow which results in respiratory infections, respiratory and cardiac failure and venous thrombosis. The incidence of accidents in the home and on the roads is increased.

Calorie intake

Even though overeating (hyperphagia) is occasionally associated with obesity, the majority of fat people do not eat too much. The adage 'fat comes from food' is misleading. Many well-carried out studies of food intake by obese and non-obese children and adults showed a similar energy content in the daily diet; some trials even demonstrated a *lower* calorie intake by obese subjects[27].

When lean subjects increase their calorie intake, obesity does not automatically result. In 1902 R. O. Neuman found that his bodyweight remained constant during a three-year experiment during which he increased his energy uptake in three steps from 1766 to 2403 kcals/day (7417 to 10 093 kJ/day). His interpretation that the excess food was used to produce increased amounts of heat (luxuconsumption) has in recent years been substantiated[27]. Obese subjects, however, appear to produce a lower thermo-

IDEAL WEIGHT TABLE

Men of 25 years and over (in indoor clothing)

Height (in shoes)		Small frame		Medium frame		Large frame	
ft in	(cm)	lb	kg	lb	kg	lb	kg
5 1	(155)	112–120	(51–54)	118–129	(54–59)	126–141	(57–64)
5 2	(157)	115–123	(52–56)	121–133	(55–60)	129–144	(59–65)
5 3	(160)	118–126	(54–57)	124–136	(56–62)	132–148	(60–67)
5 4	(163)	121–129	(55–58)	127–139	(58–63)	135–152	(61–69)
5 5	(165)	124–133	(56–60)	130–143	(59–65)	138–156	(63–71)
5 6	(168)	128–137	(58–62)	134–147	(61–67)	142–161	(64–73)
5 7	(170)	132–141	(60–64)	138–152	(63–69)	147–166	(67–75)
5 8	(173)	136–145	(62–66)	142–156	(64–71)	151–170	(68–77)
5 9	(175)	140–150	(63–68)	146–160	(66–73)	155–174	(70–79)
5 10	(178)	144–154	(65–70)	150–165	(68–75)	159–179	(72–81)
5 11	(180)	148–158	(67–72)	154–170	(70–77)	164–184	(74–83)
6 0	(183)	152–162	(69–74)	158–175	(72–80)	168–189	(76–86)
6 1	(185)	156–167	(71–76)	162–180	(74–82)	173–194	(78–88)
6 2	(188)	160–171	(73–78)	167–185	(76–84)	178–199	(81–90)
6 3	(190)	164–175	(74–80)	172–190	(78–86)	182–204	(83–92)

Women aged 25 and over (in indoor clothing)

ft in	(cm)	lb	kg	lb	kg	lb	kg
4 8	(142)	92–98	(42–44)	96–107	(44–49)	104–119	(47–54)
4 9	(145)	94–101	(43–46)	98–110	(45–50)	106–122	(48–55)
4 10	(147)	96–104	(44–47)	101–113	(46–51)	109–125	(48–57)
4 11	(150)	99–107	(45–48)	104–116	(47–53)	112–128	(51–58)
5 0	(152)	102–110	(46–50)	107–119	(48–54)	115–131	(52–59)
5 1	(155)	105–113	(48–51)	110–122	(50–55)	118–134	(53–60)
5 2	(157)	108–116	(49–53)	113–126	(51–57)	121–138	(55–63)
5 3	(160)	111–119	(50–54)	116–130	(53–59)	125–142	(57–64)
5 4	(163)	114–123	(52–56)	120–135	(54–61)	129–146	(58–66)
5 5	(165)	118–127	(53–58)	124–139	(56–63)	133–150	(60–68)
5 6	(168)	122–131	(55–59)	128–143	(58–65)	137–154	(62–70)
5 7	(170)	126–135	(57–61)	132–147	(60–67)	141–158	(64–72)
5 8	(173)	130–140	(59–63)	136–151	(62–69)	145–163	(66–74)
5 9	(175)	134–144	(61–65)	140–155	(63–70)	149–168	(68–76)
5 10	(178)	138–148	(63–67)	144–159	(65–72)	153–173	(69–78)

(For women aged between 18 and 25 substract 1 lb (½ kg) for each year under 25)

genic response when they overeat and thus, even when made lean by dieting, show a lower luxuconsumption after eating and therefore gain weight readily even with a modest dietary increase. It had been suggested that obese or potentially obese individuals are particularly vulnerable to dietary fat.

Basal metabolic rate (BMR)

A fundamental question is whether fat subjects have a lower BMR than leaner individuals. This is difficult to ascertain in the obese, because the increased bulk of the tissues itself raises the BMR – due to increased biochemical synthetic activity and other energy-dependent processes carried out by cells. However, when obese people are made lean by dieting their BMR has been shown to be significantly lower than that of spontaneously slim matched controls.

Animals that adapt to cold or to increased dietary energy intake by an enhancement of heat production appear to do so by hypertrophy of their brown fat, found in man in the adipose tissue of the back in the paravertebral and perirenal regions. This form of adipose tissue is rich in mitochondria which can produce heat energy by the oxidation of triglycerides and fatty acids, but which have a poor capacity to use energy to synthesize fats and other large molecules. In this adipose tissue, heat production is stimulated by both noradrenaline and ephedrine. There is suggestive evidence that obese people are deficient in brown fat and this is the physiological basis for their poor thermogenic response to food[28].

Movement and obesity

Gross obesity predisposes to inactivity. However, in these individuals movement requires a greater expenditure of energy than in thin people. There is no evidence that fat people utilize less energy in physical activity. Some studies on obese children indicated that they perform less vigorous movements compared with thin children involved in the same type of activity[28]; but, the greater effort in propelling a heavy body could more than compensate for sluggishness of movement.

Causes of obesity

The cause of common obesity is not known. It is not likely that one-fifth of the population has a defect in brown fat which causes obesity. However, over the last century physical activity has declined in the West. At the same time commercial interests have grown to promote the consumption of high-calorie foods, which has resulted in the seductive advertising, presentation and flavouring of foods. Whereas the majority of the population can adjust to the increase in calorie consumption and decrease in physical activity by an augmentation in heat production, about 20 per cent cannot adapt in this way and so become fat.

General management of obesity

Many social and psychological difficulties can arise in obesity. The subject is exposed to demonstrations of disgust or amusement in others. Buying clothes is a humiliating procedure – either the appropriate size is not available, or if it is, styles are dowdy or grotesque. Walking upstairs, crossing the road, fitting into buses and trains and getting into lifts can be difficult, and any physical activity can produce copious sweating. Job employment may also be restricted. Both the patient and his doctor develop a sense of hopelessness. These patients suffer a high incidence of depressive illness, anxiety neurosis and low self-esteem.

Exercise Although the condition is not usually primarily due to excessive eating combined with inactivity, weight loss will occur if physical activity is increased and dietary energy content is reduced. Apart from the calorie expenditure during the exercise, a prolonged bout of rigorous exercise is followed by a phase of accelerated metabolism which can persist for a further one or two days. Before exercise is undertaken, medical conditions which could make this undesirable should be eliminated. However, even with angina pectoris a closely supervised progressive programme of exercises can improve both exercise tolerance and the patient's confidence and sense of wellbeing.

In the young, healthy, mildly to moderately obese subject, for exercise to make any impact at all, a minimum of thirty minutes' daily exercise of sufficient severity to produce breathlessness is required. Those whose profession dictates that they stay slim, such as actors and models, usually find considerably more exercise is needed; for example, two one-hour schedules daily are not unusual. But not many people persist in such exacting regimes if their livelihood does not depend on it.

Diet The other side of the equation is diet. The difficulties involved in modifying a person's diet are even greater than changing his level of physical activity. The relationship between an individual and his diet has been described as so complex as to defy analysis. And a similarly complex collection of factors must exist between a person's body image and the efforts he or she may make to modify their appearance.

The long-term outcome of severe dietary restriction is poor. If treatment has to be carried out in hospital, it is very unlikely that the diet will be sustained afterwards. It is probably more realistic to prescribe initially a 2000-kcal (8400-kJ) diet and only reduce this if, with no defaulting, no weight is lost. It is much more realistic to aim at long-term small losses in weight with concomitant dietary re-education, than to lose 1 kg weekly for a short period. Besides, with strict calorie restriction, the initial loss is water (due to the low salt content in a minimal diet) and in lean body mass (such as muscle). A slower weight loss depletes fatty stores with less change in lean tissues.

The initial step is to establish the principles of a measured calorie diet. The most successful of these incorporate a broad range of foodstuffs. Starch-containing foods are included, but high-fat items are severely restricted. A list of banned items (such as chocolate and cakes) includes food of high-fat, sugar and energy content. Eating must be only at meal times and nibbling between meals should be forbidden. Meals should only take place in certain rooms, preferably with other people, and three or four times a day – many obese people eat only in the evenings.

Maintaining a diet Although most patients who start an energy-restricted diet do not maintain it beyond three months, frequent consultations with their physicians may help prolong the effort. These consultations seem to be most effective when held at two- to three-weekly intervals. At these sessions there is no question of the physician adopting a critical or punitive attitude to dietary lapses, but it is helpful for the patient to keep a detailed diary of his daily diet and exercise. Circumstances associated with failures to comply with the regime should be noted and discussed. In a proportion of individuals eating may be a response to anxiety, depression or other feelings of dissatisfaction. The awareness of this reaction may greatly assist re-education of eating behaviour, and underlines the need to consider that only hunger is an appropriate signal for eating. In those subjects who do adopt a regular exercise programme, its reward is not only the feeling of wellbeing and improved body appearance, but the ability to increase the calorie content of the diet and yet maintain weight loss.

Psychotherapy Many of the studies on the effects of psychotherapy and behavioural therapy on obesity show no association with successful weight reduction in the long term[28].

Group therapy is used with some success in the short and medium term for the treatment of obesity. Weight Watchers is a popular group therapy and does produce good results as long as the individual attends meetings. Long-term results, though, are disappointing after leaving the group.

Case history: losing weight with the help of group therapy

Mrs T. D., aged thirty-eight, had been obese since adolescence but after the birth of each of her four children gained progressively more weight. At a height of 5 ft 6in (1.7 m) and weight of 12½ st (78 kg) she joined a group which helped her maintain a low-calorie diet (1000 kcal/4200 kJ per day) until she had lost 14 lb (6 kg). The diet was then made less severe but still restricted in calories and particularly low in carbohydrate. An exercise program was started but not maintained beyond six months. Nevertheless, while belonging to the group she lost weight and after three years she weighed 10st 4 lb (63 kg). Two years after leaving the group her weight is 11½ st (72 kg) which she manages to maintain despite occasional binges.

The majority of obese individuals who lose weight by dieting do not keep their weight loss. Within three years over 80 per cent are back to their former state. However, some strong-willed and highly motivated patients do permanently alter their eating habits and stay lean.

Massive obesity

Massive obesity (that is, over twice ideal body weight) is possibly more often associated with overeating than less severe forms of the condition, but the evidence for this is inadequate. As with other forms of obesity, a sufficiently low-energy diet will cause weight loss. However, it would take one to two years for a patient to lose 110 lb (50 kg) at 1.1–2.2 lb (0.5–1 kg) loss/week, even if he could persist on a daily deficit of 1000 kcal (4200 kJ). Even after a myocardial infarction few patients diet at this level of deprivation for more than three months.

Exercise can be useful, but in massively obese patients the incidence of hypertension and coronary artery disease is high and correspondingly increases the hazards of embarking on vigorous exercise. More gentle and graded exercise is appropriate but less energy is consumed.

Special procedures in management

Dental splinting is effective and is maintained up to nine months at a time, but weight is rapidly gained when the wiring is removed.

Surgical procedures Effective surgical procedures include:

- Vagotomy
- Gastric pouch production
- Gastric partition
- Gastric bypass
- Intestinal bypass – leaving less than 20 in (50 cm) of small intestine in continuity
- Biliopancreatic and biliointestinal bypass.

All the above procedures, though hazardous, produce significant weight loss, often more than 30 per cent of body weight. Surprisingly the weight loss is not mainly due to malabsorption but in most cases due to eating less. This is partly mechanical (as in the case of gastric operations and vagotomy), due to the stomach filling and becoming distended rapidly, but mainly due to alterations in gastrointestinal hormone release. Cholecystokin-pancreozymin (CCK-PZ), for example, is thought to be a satiety hormone which, apart from local gut effects, enters the brain and signals a disinclination to continue eating.

Such operations are carried out on patients weighing less than 330 lb (150 kg) – so that the postoperative weight would be less than 220 lb (100 kg) – and in those under the age of fifty.

Non-drug treatment plans in obesity

The patient should visit the physician each week for weighing and discussion of the programme. For the first two weeks, no diet or extra exercise is stipulated, but the subject should keep a note book and record everything eaten. At the next visit the sole modification to diet should be only to eat at mealtimes and sitting at a table – no snacks, no interim nibbling, no eating during other activities.

These measures may themselves cause significant weight loss, but if a diet is required this can be applied in two stages:

1. Eliminate calorie-concentrated foods (sweets, chocolates, cakes, pastry and pies, fried food, cream) and substitute with high-fibre food. Although the physician should not strive too hard to alter the ratio of carbohydrate, protein and fat which the patient enjoys, there is some evidence that a decrease in fat and an increase in carbohydrate is preferable. Thus, do not reduce carbohydrates, but encourage the eating of foods containing complex carbohydrates, such as bread, potatoes, beans, pasta and rice. Simple sugars, however, should be greatly reduced.

2. If necessary give detailed instructions about a calorie-restricted diet. The usual energy requirements of the patient should be assessed and a 500-kcal (2100-kJ) deficit prescribed. This cannot usually be maintained beyond four weeks, so at this time a relaxation back to the first stage ought to be made.

   Exercise, if sustained beyond thirty minutes and carried out sufficiently vigorously each day, will also help weight loss.

THE USE OF DRUGS IN OBESITY

Drugs play only a minor role in the treatment of obesity. On their own, without dietary measures, they are useless and potentially harmful.

The stimulant drugs are contraindicated in patients with cardiovascular disease (particularly hypertension and ischaemic heart disease) and in subjects with a history of manic-depressive illness, schizophrenia and drug abuse. They must not be given to patients taking MAOIs.

The stimulant drugs must only be used to help a motivated patient to suffer a 500–1000 kcal (2100–4200 kJ) daily diet over a prolonged period. Surprisingly, these drugs can provide assistance for over six months, and naturally must be stopped if the diet is abandoned. If the diet is adhered to the patient will lose 1–2 lb 4 oz (0.5–1.0 kg) each week. A critical time is when the drug is stopped and the patient encouraged to maintain a modified and less severe diet with a change in eating habits. The usual pattern is that patients who have satisfactorily lost weight with anorectic drugs, gain weight when the drugs are stopped.

Drugs used to curtail eating are:

- Anorectic agents
- Bulk-increasing agents

ANORECTIC AGENTS

Anorectic agents include the following.

- Fenfluramine
- Amphetamine } should *not* be used for obesity
- Phenmetrazine }
- Diethylpropion
- Phentermine
- Mazindol

Fenfluramine

Drugs such as cyproheptadine and pizotifen which block 5-HT receptors usually increase appetite. Fenfluramine potentiates the release of 5-HT into brain synapses and simultaneously blocks its removal by neuronal reuptake. Unlike other anorectic drugs, fenfluramine is not a central nervous system stimulant. An additional action is that it may potentiate the utilization of glucose by muscle cells. It has been suggested that because of this action it may be of value in treating obese diabetics.

Side-effects Fenfluramine can produce nausea and diarrhoea. Commonly sedation, fatigue and somnolence develop. Sometimes nightmares and disturbed sleep result, particularly in patients who are depressed or have a past history of depression. The appearance of nightmares may indicate that an episode of depression is developing due to the drug. Depression may not only occur during treatment but can also appear on abrupt withdrawal of the drug. The action of antihypertensive drugs may be antagonized and the effects of sedatives potentiated.

Excessive doses are dangerous and successful suicide is not uncommon with this drug. Toxic psychosis (with delirium, delusions and hallucinations) may be followed by fits and coma. Early features of overdose include abdominal pain, nausea, vomiting and cardiac tachyarrhythmias. These may be followed by rotatory nystagmus and hyperpyrexia.

Dose The initial dose of fenfluramine is 20 mg twice daily. If this dose is tolerated and a greater anorectic effect is needed, each dose may be increased each week by 20 mg up to a maximum daily dose of 120 mg. At the end of the period of treatment the dose should similarly be reduced in a stepwise fashion.

Ponderax PA capsules (60 mg) are a sustained-action presentation. The dose is 1–2 capsules daily.

Amphetamine and phenmetrazine

These are indirectly acting sympathomimetic drugs which have a stimulatory action on the brain by displacing noradrenaline and dopamine from vesicular stores. Initially they decrease appetite but some tolerance to this effect can develop. Nevertheless, those who abuse these drugs for long periods do tend to continue to eat poorly and lose weight. Large doses can produce a paranoid reaction and auditory hallucinations. A full-blown and sustained schizophrenic episode may develop – particularly in a person with a history of schizophrenia – but this can occur in any individual.

High doses can precipitate hypertensive episodes, cardiac arrhythmias and fits. Withdrawal of these drugs can cause somnolence, depression and hyperphagia.

Such central nervous system stimulants readily produce dependence and should not be used as anorectic agents.

Diethylpropion

This has a similar action to amphetamine in that it is a central nervous system stimulant and can produce feelings of anxiety and tremulousness, dry mouth and insomnia. However, the dependence risk is said to be less than with amphetamine and phenmetrazine[18].

Dependence can develop with diethylpropion, as can depression on withdrawal, but these are probably less readily caused than with amphetamine and are possibly less severe when they do occur.

Dose The usual dose of diethylpropion is 50–75 mg daily, as a single morning dose or in divided doses. Tenuate Dospan is a sustained-action tablet containing 75 mg of diethylpropion hydrochloride. One tablet is swallowed mid-morning.

Phentermine

This has similar properties and dangers to diethylpropion.

Duromine is a sustained-release capsule and Ionamin is a capsule of resin-bound drug. Both are available in two sizes, 15 and 30 mg.

Dose The daily dose is a single capsule of either size.

Mazindol

This is another central nervous system stimulant which has anorectic properties. Like the other drugs it can produce nervousness, tremulousness and insomnia. In some individuals paradoxical sedation may occur.

Dose The dose is 2 mg taken after breakfast.

BULK-INCREASING AGENTS

An increase in dietary fibre by encouraging the incorporation of high-residue foods such as wholewheat bread, whole potatoes and legumes does not in itself result in a reduction in daily calorie intake, but in the motivated patient helps to avoid eating highly concentrated energy-laden foods. Also the high-fibre foods usually involve more prolonged chewing than high calorie items and in this way provide a greater degree of oral gratification. They do not provide a stimulus for early cutoff (that is, satiety) during a meal.

Effects

Methylcellulose and Prefil (sterculia 55 per cent plus guar gum 5 per cent as granules) are swallowed with water so that these non-digested substances swell and theoretically produce feelings of fullness. Another possible effect of these substances is to impair absorption of energy-containing foodstuffs.

Bran does not inhibit the absorption of lipids and sugars, but legume fibre and guar gum appear to inhibit absorption of glucose and possibly lipids. For the treatment of overweight patients, though, this effect is negligible[18].

ANOREXIA NERVOSA

Anorexia nervosa is a psychiatric syndrome of unknown cause, with females being affected more often than males in a ratio of 20:1. The commonest age of onset is thirteen to eighteen years, but the condition can start at any time in adult life. Depressive illness, anxiety states, puberty, parturition and recent marriage are illnesses and life events frequently associated with onset of the condition and may therefore possibly play a causative role.

The psychoanalytical view of the illness is that the patient starves herself or induces vomiting or takes purgatives because she has a fear of becoming fat. She produces a distorted body image in which a body weight of, say, 70–90 per cent of ideal is thought to be swollen, gross and grotesque. The analytical reason for this distortion is a terror of growing up with its concomitant loss of a dependent relationship with parents (or husband) and the assumption of adult responsibilities. The overlying symbolism of not eating, vomiting and purgation is said to represent non-acceptance and rejection. The secondary gains of the syndrome are not joining in family life (as symbolized by eating together), becoming the focus of attention (in a manipulative childlike way) and amenorrhoea (thus childlike and cannot become pregnant). Even physicians who do not think in psychoanalytical terms must come to terms with the fact that this condition leads to death by starvation.

GENERAL MANAGEMENT OF ANOREXIA

Home management

Some anorectics can be treated on an outpatient basis. This group includes those whose disease has lasted for less than a year and whose weight loss and general condition do not appear to be life-threatening.

During the early consultations at least, the doctor should see the patient's close relatives (especially parents or spouse) as well as having personal interviews with the patient. It is helpful to assess the stability of the home and to try to identify any potentially treatable sources of domestic tension.

The most important aim of the initial consultation is not to enter into a conflict with the patient, but to explain that her anxieties about obesity and conflict about eating are understood.

Achieving a target weight The next step at this stage is to draw a chart with the patient's present weight and her target weight on it. The target should be discussed with the patient and a figure agreed on. Usually somewhere between 85 and 100 per cent of ideal weight is found acceptable. A rate of increase of weight is then chosen and this is drawn onto the chart; 1–2 lb 4 oz (0.5–1 kg)/week would be a satisfactory rate.

The next decision to be taken by doctor and patient is the method by which this should be attained. Forced vomiting and purgation should be enquired about, noted sympathetically, and then either stopped or arrangements made for admission to hospital. The patient should be told that eating is to be carried out in the normal social setting – with the family – and a diet schedule chosen. At first very small meals may be allowed but within three weeks a daily intake of 3000–4000 kcal (12600–16800 kJ) is quite possible. Secret binges (followed by guilt and depression) should stop as soon as the patient stops feeling hungry.

Visits to the doctor every week to ten days allow weighing, filling in actual weight on the chart and discussions of how close this is to the target weight for that visit. If the patient can be persuaded to keep an accurate diary of dietary intake and external events, it may be possible to show an effect of emotional distress on diet and weight.

Even at the early stages of treatment it should be explained to patient and family that failure of treatment at home will necessitate admission to a specialized unit.

Case history: weight gain on a high-calorie diet with regular follow-up

A nurse aged eighteen gave a weight of 7 st 2 lb (44 kg) when filling in her health form six months before starting training at a London teaching hospital. The letter from her family doctor said that she had suffered from an episode of anorexia when she was sixteen but had had no trouble since.

On starting at nursing school she was weighed by the physician in the nurses health service. Her weight was actually 6 st 4 lb (39 kg), height 5 ft 2 in (1.5 m) and she had had amenorrhoea for the past eighteen months. She did not admit the purgation or forced vomiting but did say she sometimes ate excessively and felt guilty afterwards. For the previous few months she had worried about losing weight and the difficulty she had in eating with others.

She was asked to attend the clinic at weekly intervals and a 3500 kcal (14700 kJ) diet was explained to her. These measures alone resulted in a gain in weight of about 1 lb (0.5 kg) each week until she weighed 7 st 9 lb (48 kg), at which time she began to menstruate again.

Inpatient management

The patient remains in hospital until a high-calorie diet is being consumed without any external persuasion, good health is restored and ideal weight has been attained and maintained for two to three weeks.

On admission, as at home, a chart of real and ideal progress is plotted. The weight is measured every day before breakfast.

In many units a scheme of rewards is used. A series of subtargets based on weight gains of 2 lb 4 oz–4 lb 8 oz (1–2 kg) per week are decided on, and the attainment of each of these is rewarded by: abandonment of being totally confined to bed; being allowed to go to the lavatory, have a bath, wear normal clothing, go out to the cinema, and to have weekends at home – and many variations of these. Initially visiting is *not* allowed, and this alone seems to produce a reduction in emotional tension in both the patient and her family.

Much depends on the quality of the nursing staff. A calm and steady approach eventually wins round the majority of militant non-eaters. Similarly, close supervision, experience and tact are needed to detect and dissuade secret vomiters and purgative abusers. The practitioner plays a vital role after discharge from hospital. The patient may be seen initially every two weeks, and if improvement is maintained, the visits can then be spaced out further.

Severe cases Some patients require tube-feeding initially, and intravenous supplementation (as in severe hypokalaemia) may be necessary. Severely emaciated patients who have semistarved themselves for a year or more may not be able to take solid food by mouth and are given a liquid diet in small amounts at two-hourly intervals.

ECT and psychosurgery are rarely used and are reserved for very severely affected patients as a life-saving measure, or if the condition is long-standing and other forms of treatment have failed.

After restoration of weight has commenced, psychiatric counselling is undertaken with the patient and also parents or spouse. In other words, more than one member of the family may become identified as patients.

DRUG TREATMENT IN ANOREXIA

Drugs do not play a major role in the treatment of anorexia, but in some patients they have proved to be very valuable.

Drugs used in anorexia

- 5-HT antagonists
- Neuroleptics
- Antidepressants
- Anxiolytics
- Hypoglycaemic agents (now not used)

5-hydroxytryptamine (5-HT) antagonists

Blockers of 5-hydroxytryptamine receptors, such as cyproheptadine and pizotifen, increase the appetite and in many subjects cause a gain in weight.

Cyproheptadine This is an antagonist of 5-HT and H_1 histamine receptors. It is mainly used as an antiallergic agent, but its disadvantages for this purpose include sedation and increased appetite.

The recommended dose is 4 mg four times a day. Such frequent administration is probably not required in anorexia, particularly as the drug is sedating. Perhaps a single evening dose of 4 mg should be tried initially and increased to 4 mg morning and evening if the starting dose has no effect. The action of other sedatives (such as anxiolytics, neuroleptics or antidepressants) will be greatly increased and could amount to a dangerous interaction.

Neuroleptics

Chlorpromazine is sometimes used in anorexia. Any sedative can increase the appetite, but the neuroleptics are particularly powerful in this respect. An added effect of chlorpromazine is that it reduces feelings of tension and panic and thus reduces the drama and conflict of mealtimes.

Although large doses (for example, 500 mg daily) of chlorpromazine have been used, if the drug is to be tried in a patient it is desirable to start with a much lower dose, such as 10–25 mg before meals. Epilepsy is one toxic effect particularly associated with this method of treatment.

Antidepressants

Antidepressants are indicated for anorectic patients suffering from overt depression, but some anxious and agitated patients will also respond to these drugs. Amitriptyline in low doses (for example 75 mg) given at night is usually satisfactory.

MAOIs are rarely used.

Anxiolytics

The benzodiazepines often increase the appetite of non-anorectic individuals and cause a gain in weight, but they do not usually have this effect in anorexia nervosa. However, they are sometimes used when a patient is admitted to hospital if major conflict arises at mealtimes and panic states occur.

Hypoglycaemic agents

In the past, severe intractable anorexia was treated with very small doses of insulin given ten to fifteen minutes before meals. Although this measure does increase the appetite, there is a danger of severe hypoglycaemia with convulsions and brain damage. Hypoglycaemic agents cannot therefore be recommended, and should be considered as contraindicated in anorexia nervosa.

PRACTICAL POINTS

Obesity

- In the treatment of obesity the patient should visit the physician each week for weighing and discussion of the programme.
- A two-stage diet should be inaugurated, together with a vigorous programme of daily exercise.

Anorexia nervosa

- In the treatment of anorexia nervosa the patient should visit her physician for a sympathetic discussion of agreed target weights.
- Very small meals taken with the family are allowed for anorectics, afterwards being increased to 3000–4000 kcal (12600–16800 kJ) per day.

11
Physical and psychological interactions

BACKGROUND

In clinical medicine there are many examples of associations between physical and psychiatric disturbances. These can loosely be classified as follows:

1. Physical illnesses causing psychological disturbances due to the mental stress of the primary illness. Such reactions include depression or anxiety in response to pain, loss of function or fear of disfiguration.
2. Physical illness producing mental disturbances because of individual susceptibility. For example, patients with early senile dementia may show no clinical abnormality until a physical disturbance such as fever or the use of sedatives precipitates an acute confusional state.
3. Physical illnesses such as hypoglycaemia, uraemia and myxoedema usually produce both physical and psychiatric symptoms and signs. Similarly some chemical substances – in particular psychotropic drugs and alcohol – frequently cause both physical and mental toxic effects.
4. There is a large group of physical illnesses, the course of which may be influenced by psychological factors. Although asthma, ulcerative colitis and peptic ulcer are among those singled out as being typical members of this group of psychosomatic illnesses, enthusiasts would consider that there could be a psychological component in the causation of all physical illness. However, there does seem to be more evidence of non-physical causes in migraine (see Chapter 12) and spastic colon than in cancer, for instance. Nevertheless the field is constantly changing. For example, some patients with migraine may be cured by omitting chocolate or oranges from their diet, and some who have suffered from spastic colon all their lives can experience permanent relief on introducing bran to their diet. On the other hand, there is some evidence that cancer may be more common in depressives and in people who have experienced other forms of grief and loss and other forms of physical or psychological trauma. There are, however, many clearcut examples of physical symptoms – in

particular pain – which are expressions of mental anguish, as frequently occurs in pathological and unresolved mourning.
5. Physical signs which are a manifestation of a psychological disturbance, e.g. tics.

PSYCHOLOGICAL RESPONSES TO PHYSICAL ILLNESS

Although it is convenient to describe the psychological and physical components of illness as distinct from each other, in disease they form a single entity. Depression, for example, may form a part of the condition – as in brucellosis, influenza and rheumatoid arthritis. It is also possible that emotional responses may determine the course of the illness – the mental reaction to bodily illness is influenced by the patient's personality. Dependent, inadequate individuals may welcome the illness and attempt to prolong and deepen the dependency state. Obsessional patients may be particularly distressed by the break from routine, but may experience further suffering if the nature of the illness or treatment is not fully discussed by the physician.

Emotional reactions

The emotional reactions to pain show much individual variation[29]. The very young and old, and the anxious and depressed appear to experience more distress from painful illness. As measured on the Eysenck Personality Inventory those who experience more pain but do not complain have higher neuroticism and lower extroversion scores than patients who complain or who do not experience pain, when comparing a group of sufferers from the same condition.

A physical illness which is neither severe nor painful may sometimes produce serious psychiatric illness if the physical change produced has important personal significance to the patient. Thus a skin lesion – especially on the face or hands – impairment of athletic ability, modification of employability, alteration in the voice or impairment of the sense of smell could be profoundly important to some individuals. On the other hand, a real threat to life – particularly if laced with much uncertainty about future recurrence (as with a myocardial infarction) – will distress the majority of patients.

Psychiatric complications

The commonest psychiatric complication of physical illness is depression, but anxiety is also common, particularly in the early stages of a serious illness.

Phobic anxiety may also develop, particularly in relation to a specific procedure (such as venepuncture) or therapy (such as a drug). Depression during convalescence can be accompanied by hypochondriasis which may actually delay recovery and rehabilitation. Such problems during recovery from a physical illness carry an increased risk of suicide. Depression following a myocardial infarction can result in the patient never resuming his work. Some physicians suspect that depression predisposes to reinfarction[30].

Other psychotic reactions such as mania and paranoia are less common. However, loss of sight or of hearing may precipitate a paranoid illness. In the elderly loss of a special sense can precipitate an acute confusional episode.

What to do

Much anxiety can be prevented by the physician giving a full explanation of the illness, its likely progress and its treatment. Every opportunity must be given to the patient to ask questions (and go over old explanations). The direction and intensity of the patient's questions provide an indication of how much or how little the patient wants to know.

Individual circumstances will affect the management of convalescence. In those for whom the physical illness has produced some secondary gain – such as financial compensation, or escape from unhappiness at work or home, or the opportunity to alter a marital relationship by becoming passive and dependent – recovery may be considerably delayed.

PSYCHOSOMATIC ILLNESS

Antecedent factors

Significant life events appear to act as triggers for the appearance of physical illness, or for the patient to seek medical help for a longstanding physical complaint. Some events are particularly stressful. T. H. Holmes and R. H. Rahe produced a scale representing the impact of various stress-provoking situations by observing how often this provoked breakdown[31].

Stress-provoking situations (from a list published in the New York Times, 10 June 1973)

Event	Scale of impact
Death of spouse	100
Divorce	73
Marital separation	65
Marriage	50
Marital reconciliation	45
Retirement	45
Sexual difficulties	39
Change in financial state	38
Taking out a moderately large mortgage	31
Change of responsibilities at work	29
Child leaving home	29
Outstanding personal achievement	28
Beginning or end of school	26
Change in sleeping habits	16
Change in eating habits	15
Going on holiday	13
Christmas	12

Of course, not all these stresses can immediately be recognized as unpleasant. Not everyone becomes ill when confronted with the necessity to change and adjust to life events. In fact in any population a small proportion of people account for a large proportion of the illness; some people appear to be prone to various conditions or accidents or symptoms.

Certain schools of psychoanalytical thought go even further and relate particular personalities to individual psychosomatic illnesses. Thus the rigid obsessional personality is prone to coronary heart disease (see below), and migraine, particularly just after the resolution of a tension (see Chapter 12). Patients with peptic ulcer have been pushed by life into positions of leadership and responsibility even though they are basically passive and dependent – the hypersecretion of gastric acid and pepsin being a physical expression of preparation for passively receiving food. Asthma is described as a way of expressing depression due to not receiving enough love from parents; the asthmatic wheeze is a cry for love to a mother who is withholding this from the patient. Hypertension, on the other hand, may be considered as the visceral component of sympathetic nervous system activity – without the outward manifestations of fight, flight or fright. The psychoanalytical description of the cause of hypertension may in this way be due to conflicts arising from poorly expressed aggression. Similarly, eczema and other skin conditions are related to conflicts regarding exhibitionism. Colitis has been described as representing conflicts relating to learning bowel control.

Such statements are not universally accepted in medicine – mainly because these concepts do not readily lend themselves to experimental testing.

PSYCHOLOGICAL FACTORS IN CORONARY ARTERY DISEASE

Coronary artery disease is a major cause of death and disability in middle age. Some risk factors have been identified, including smoking, lack of physical exercise, diet and hypertension. The incidence in coronary artery disease has in recent years fallen in the United States, but risen in some parts of western Europe. There is no convincing evidence that changes in the risk factors mentioned above have been the sole reason for the changing incidence in heart disease. In particular, this condition is relatively uncommon in Japan but has become increasingly common in Japanese living abroad – even in those with no change in eating and smoking habits.

Psychological factors have been postulated as contributing to the development of coronary disease and to the timing of a myocardial infarction[32, 33].

Type A behaviour

Attention has been called to the so-called type A behaviour which may be linked with proneness to coronary disease. Type A individuals are overconscientious, rigid workaholics, oppressed by deadlines which they feel duty-bound to meet at all costs. The coronary personality (which is claimed to be the type A personality) is not impulsive and accident prone but usually takes considered action, is competitive and constantly tries to seize authority. In short, he is striving, ambitious and authority-seeking.

Life changes

In addition there is evidence that life changes – particularly those which reduce feelings of security or lower self-esteem – are followed by increased risk of physical disease. Widows have a significantly raised risk of cardiovascular (and other) disease during the five years after bereavement. A series of men who had recently suffered a myocardial infarction gave a history of recent divorce or loss of a close friend more frequently than in a matched control group[30, 33].

Interaction between mind and body

The mechanisms by which psychological attitudes and stresses can influence the coronary circulation are not understood. However, stresses such as public speaking and car driving can raise blood lipid and noradrenaline levels. The latter is presumably an index of general sympathetic arousal which itself results in increased platelet stickiness, raised blood pressure, increased oxygen demands by the myocardium and proneness to cardiac arrhythmias.

Non-drug behaviour modification

It is not known whether it is possible to protect individuals from stressful life events or whether type A behaviour can be modified. Certainly a warm and closely knit family life can provide much support against the stresses of external change. A cultural pattern of a strictly hierarchical society – as occurs in Japanese families and work organizations – is also protective. The possibility of behaviour modification by group and individual therapy is being investigated[30, 33]. Even if this is effective, it is important to aim for lifelong alteration in psychological reactions. It is not yet known if behaviour modification will, in fact, result in a reduction in the incidence of ischaemic heart disease in ex-type A individuals.

Behaviour modification with drugs

Drug treatment usually plays little or no part here. The use of hypnosedatives may be counterproductive because the rebound increase in disturbing vivid dreams with multiple wakenings (REM rebound) may precipitate episodes of myocardial ischaemia. However, the prophylactic use of beta-blockers in patients who have already experienced a myocardial infarction may reduce the manifestations of heightened sympathetic drive.

The intensely anxiety-provoking nature of coronary care units can best be reduced by intelligent, sensitive and perceptive staff. Failing that (or even in addition to such care) large doses of a benzodiazepine may help over the short period that a patient is in intensive care.

PAIN, SYMPATHETIC AROUSAL AND HYPERVENTILATION

These may arise separately, but frequently are present together in different degrees. In tense, anxious individuals, an increase in muscle tension is a physical expression of perceiving the environment as hostile and dangerous. The patient is preparing himself for the next threat. Continuously contracted muscles soon begin to ache, and the subject then finds the pain produces more stress and a threat to wellbeing. Very often the patient is not aware of his global tenseness but only of his pain. Any muscle group can be involved, but it is most commonly the frontalis, occipital, neck and back muscles. Tension in the forehead is a common cause of frontal headache, and in adults or children may produce the physical sign of vertical furrowing between the brows. Other physical conditions such as sinusitis or cervical spondylosis can further trigger and aggravate this tension-induced muscular pain.

Some degree of hyperventilation accompanies any form of anxiety-provoked muscle tension. However, prolonged hyperventilation can produce paraesthesiae, tetany and cerebral vasoconstriction – the latter possibly leading to light-headedness, giddiness and fainting. Bronchoconstriction can also be provoked, particularly in asthmatics. Other features of sympathetic arousal that may arise include sweating, palpitations and tremor.

Management

The management of this group of conditions must start with making an accurate diagnosis. Serious physical illness (such as tuberculosis) can present as anxiety and/or depression. If the condition is primarily that of anxiety, it is important to reassure the patient that there is in fact no sinister underlying disorder.

The next critical stage is not to distress the patient by implying he is imagining the illness or is malingering. Pain is never a physical sign but is always subjective in whatever level of the body it arises.

If the patient is depressed the use of antidepressants may be helpful. However, use of anxiolytics or beta-blockers may not be at all useful, and even when these are used with success they have troublesome toxicity and can only be used for limited periods.

Apart from listening, discussion and explanation, the most valuable forms of treatment are muscular relaxation techniques and the practice of controlled relaxed and prolonged breathing exercises. Other methods of relaxation which do not have the hazards of drugs include biofeedback, meditation, yoga and hypnosis. Audio tapes and records and books are available to help with muscular and mental relaxation procedures[33].

FUNCTIONAL DISORDERS OF THE INTESTINAL TRACT

Before the diagnosis of a functional disorder of any part of the alimentary tract can be made, it is essential to exclude the presence of organic disease. Thus in order to diagnose the irritable bowel syndrome it may be necessary to carry out routine blood tests including haematocrit and erythrocyte sedimentation rate (ESR), perform an air contrast barium enema, sigmoidoscopy and examine the faeces for blood and pathogens.

There appear to be predisposing factors in the irritable bowel syndrome: previous organic diarrhoea disease; lowered pain threshold for the colon; excessive and uncoordinated segmental contractions of the large intestine; and possibly abnormal water and electrolyte transport through the intestinal mucosa.

It is much more difficult to identify the psychological factors which might lead to this common disorder. The literature contains many uncontrolled sets of observations, which have revealed high proportions of patients with the syndrome who have depression, anxiety or marital disharmony. However, carefully carried out trials have suggested a high incidence of hysteria and depression. Psychoanalytical studies suggested that the predisposing personality is obsessional, orderly, rigid and concerned with planning and detailed organization[34].

Psychological factors can profoundly influence gastrointestinal secretion and motility. Relapses or exacerbations of the irritable bowel syndrome may follow the stresses of major life events.

Management

The management of the syndrome starts with the exclusion of organic disease – including laxative abuse and thyrotoxicosis. When the general and alimentary investigations have been found to reveal no abnormalities, it is important that the patient should not get the impression that his doctor might think that his diarrhoea and pain do not exist. The physician must reassure the patient that he understands his symptoms and explain the mechanisms by which psychological factors can affect bowel function.

Although physical treatment (such as a high-fibre diet or codeine) may produce some improvement, this varies from patient to patient, and in a single patient from time to time. The patient and his physician must resist feelings of guilt and failure if there is an exacerbation despite treatment. Support and sympathetic discussions should include the patient's spouse or other members of his family.

ASTHMA

Asthma, a condition affecting 2 to 20 per cent of the population, consists of episodes of reversible increases in airways resistance. Nevertheless, in between attacks the bronchioles continue to be hyperactive, and wheezing can be provoked by a number of factors. Despite the importance of emotional changes in precipitating asthmatic attacks, this is an example of a psychosomatic disease which can kill. Some patients may obtain benefit from procedures which reduce physical and emotional tension, but a bad attack of asthma requires vigorous drug treatment, usually with beta-agonists and steroids. To administer an anxiolytic instead is a potentially lethal mistake.

Factors that can cause asthma attacks

- Exercise
- Change in air temperature
- Sulphur dioxide
- Laughing
- Allergens
- Emotion (pleasant or unpleasant excitement)
- Respiratory infection

EPILEPSY

About half of children with cerebral palsy also have epilepsy and intellectual impairment. However, in epileptic individuals with no other motor, intellectual or sensory defect there may be psychological problems related to the epileptic phenomena or to its treatment.

Epileptic attacks

The aura of a seizure, particularly in temporal lobe epilepsy, may consist of an emotional experience such as fear or a vague feeling of unease. In psychomotor epilepsy the attack itself is often an experience of loss of contact with reality, sometimes with hallucinations of smell or other abnormality of perception. After a fit the patient usually sleeps, but some may experience other postictal psychological phenomena. Sometimes automatic unplanned behaviour occurs in which the subject behaves in a coordinated and consistent way but later has no recollection of the episode. He may resume his normal personality and find himself in an unaccustomed environment with no idea of how he arrived there. Such a pattern of illness has been used as a defence in criminal prosecution charges.

Effects of repeated fits

Repeated single fits of the grand mal or petit mal type do not usually appear to damage the brain. But if, for example, 400 petit mal absences occur each day over several years a child will suffer from the loss of accumulated experience these cause. Both intellectually and socially he will be deprived because of reduced contact with the world. Abolition of the fits by drug treatment will restore normal contact and can allow the child to catch up.

Status epilepticus is another matter. When repeated grand mal fits follow each other without regain of consciousness this amounts to a medical emergency. The patient must be admitted to a specialist unit, and even here the mortality rate is at least 10 per cent, permanent neurological and psychiatric sequelae amounting to 20 per cent. Even if the continuous fits develop in a previously healthy person (as can occur in infants with febrile convulsions) sufficient organic brain damage can result as to form a future focus for chronic epilepsy. A particularly vulnerable part of the brain for such epileptic and hypoxic injury is the temporal lobe.

Behavioural disorders associated with epilepsy

A group of behavioural disorders is said to be associated with epilepsy in some children and adolescents but it is ill-defined. In one survey one-quarter of children and one-sixth of adults with epilepsy had chronic behavioural problems, unrelated to individual fits[35]. The children may be hyperactive, moody, depressed, have angry outbursts, suffer phobias or carry out antisocial acts, all of which may be difficult to distinguish from normal adolescent behaviour. However, in some instances it is claimed that treating temporal lobe epilepsy with carbamazepine may not only reduce or abolish the fits, but act as a tranquillizer and improve the behaviour problems[35].

Psychological and sensory trigger factors

In an established epileptic, psychological factors, such as boredom, chronic frustration and unemployment, can influence the frequency of fits, and cause a deterioration. Contentment and fulfilment at home and work may produce improvement. It has been observed by some patients that even when an aura is being experienced, carrying out mental arithmetic may avert a fit. Others, though, find that mental arithmetic can trigger a fit.

Up to 6 per cent of people with epilepsy have their fits precipitated by external stimuli or particular mental activities. The most important of these are visual experiences: 20–40 per cent of epileptics have an abnormal EEG response to flickering light, and this will produce a fit during the EEG test in 2–4 per cent.

Precipitators of an epileptic fit

Visual
- Disco lights
- Television
- Sunlight shimmering on water
- Fluorescent tubes
- Metal escalators

Other sensory stimuli
- Touching a part of the body unexpectedly
- Music
- Certain smells
- Looking at particular patterns

Mental activity
- Performing music
- Reading
- Writing
- Mathematical calculations

Other sensory precipitators of a fit, and mental activity which can have a triggering effect are also shown in the table on page 139. Having to carry out discriminative mental activity under stress can also be a precipitant. Epilepsy triggered by reading is complex: in some patients this is an expression of light or pattern-induced seizures, but in others it can be because of the emotion, interest or difficulty of the material.

A fit may be followed by a reduction in emotional tension. Possibly related to this, are the rare reports of tension-relieving activities developing into epileptic precipitants. For example, a safety-pin fetishist later found that the sight of this object caused a fit, also two patients with musicogenic epilepsy had previously used loud music to relieve strong emotions.

Anticonvulsant agents

Psychological changes produced by anticonvulsant drugs are most commonly due to those agents which are usually sedating in therapeutic doses.

Phenobarbitone is a very effective anticonvulsant with a good relationship between plasma levels and fit suppression, the optimum range being 10–25 μg/ml plasma. However, this concentration is also associated with sedation and impaired motor coordination. There is a tendency for the sedation to become less with chronic treatment, but this toxic effect usually persists. Thus the intellectual and motor-skill performance of adults is impaired and children suffer the added problem of reduced learning ability in academic and social fields.

Depression may also complicate long-term treatment with phenobarbitone. Some children respond to the drug with paradoxical excitement, and they also are impaired in judgement and learning, despite being hyperactive and garrulous. Even though these children are prone to walk or even run when it would be more appropriate for them to sit still, they have poor coordination and may be ataxic. Paradoxical excitement is often an even more troublesome toxic effect than sedation.

The other major disadvantages of phenobarbitone are enzyme induction and dependence. The consequences of enzyme induction are that the dose of phenobarbitone may have to be increased in the early days of treatment and that interactions with other drugs and vitamins can occur. Thus the action of warfarin and of the contraceptive pill can be reduced, and folic acid and vitamin D destroyed more rapidly than usual. Rapid withdrawal of phenobarbitone can be followed by insomnia, panic attacks and status epilepticus.

Primidone has a reputation of producing less mental clouding, sedation and paradoxical excitement, but more ataxia than phenobarbitone. This may be unfounded because much of an administered dose of primidone is converted to phenobarbitone in the body.

Phenytoin is the drug of choice in the tonic-clonic group of epilepsies. In over 70 per cent of patients this agent on its own will prevent the majority or all of the fits. In recent years the more successful use of phenytoin monotherapy has developed

Problems associated with phenobarbitone for epileptics

- Sedation
- Impaired motor coordination
- Reduced intellectual skills in adults
- Reduced learning abilities in children
- Depression
- Paradoxical hyperactivity
- Dependence
- Enzyme induction
- Serious rebound fits on sudden withdrawal

because of the ability to measure blood levels of the drug. Optimal fit control usually corresponds to the attainment of plasma levels between 10 and 20 μg/ml. Not only is the drug highly effective, but within this range sedation and other alterations in mental function do not occur. Between 20–30 μg/ml plasma nystagmus, tremor and cerebellar ataxia may develop. In the region of 30 μg/ml and above, neurological and psychiatric toxicity may be seen, consisting of sedation, depression, paranoia and hallucinations. Rarely there is a clinical picture resembling a full-blown acute schizophrenic episode. High blood levels can be associated with severe ataxia, peripheral neuropathy, worsening of fits and coma.

It is still uncertain whether phenytoin used correctly over a long period can produce permanent effects on the intellect. There does appear to be a reduction in learning ability in epileptic children compared with controls; there is still a measurable deficit when children with other evidence of brain damage have been excluded from the series. However, at present there is no evidence that it is phenytoin (or any other drug) which is responsible for the intellectual deficit.

It is characteristically children with temporal lobe epilepsy who suffer from learning difficulties, and such educational problems may resolve in those patients who are successfully treated for epilepsy by temporal lobectomy.

Carbamazepine is probably the second drug of choice in tonic-clonic seizures. It is probably as effective as phenytoin in epilepsy but has a number of toxic effects even when correct therapeutic doses are given. Feelings of giddiness, weakness and unsteadiness are common. The drug is often sedating and this is greatly aggravated if other central depressants are given concurrently. Carbamazepine has a $t_{1/2}\beta$ of 12–20 hours after a single test dose, but it is an enzyme inducer and the $t_{1/2}\beta$ shortens in the early weeks of treatment. Thus the drug is given two or three times daily.

The sedating action is sometimes useful in epileptic children with behaviour disorders, but sedatives are not usually helpful here.

Sodium valproate is a remarkable substance which is useful in a wide range of epilepsies. It blocks gamma-aminobutyric acid (GABA) decarboxylase, thus raising the concentrations in the brain of the inhibitory neurotransmitter GABA. Sodium valproate has a half-life of 10–12 hours and is therefore given 8–12-hourly.

The drug is mildly sedating but can potentiate the sedating effects of other agents such as carbamazepine and clonazepam. It can also produce mild dyspepsia, temporary hair loss and (rarely, but particularly in children) acute hepatic necrosis.

Ethosuximide is effective only in petit mal, where it is the drug of choice. It is a remarkably non-toxic drug and its successful use in petit mal may improve a child's mental state due to alleviation of absence seizures. The drug has a $t_{1/2}\beta$ of 30–70 hours and is given once daily.

Clonazepam is a benzodiazepine specially marketed for the treatment of epilepsy. It is effective in the minor epilepsies which have in the past resisted drug treatment, including myoclonic attacks and akinetic seizures. Clonazepam can potentiate the action of sodium valproate in minor epilepsy and can be used in this combination or with ethosuximide in petit mal. Clonazepam is probably also effective in tonic-clonic fits but cannot be tolerated in long-term use in older children and adults because of sedation. Like all the benzodiazepines, anticonvulsant activity occurs with large doses which also lead to sleepiness, weakness, hypotonia, diplopia, ataxia, reduced concentration and impaired memory. Paradoxical excitement can occur, but less commonly than with the barbiturates. The benzodiazepines can induce attacks of rage, drunken-like behaviour, hypnagogic hallucinations and severe depression in some individuals.

Anticonvulsant therapy in pregnancy The risk to a woman who received anticonvulsant therapy during pregnancy of delivering a malformed infant is about one in ten. The risk of untreated epilepsy in pregnancy is probably greater than this. No anticonvulsant drug can be singled out as safe for pregnant women. The newer drugs (such as sodium valproate) have been implicated as well as the older ones (such as phenytoin).

Frequent abnormalities due to anticonvulsant therapy in pregnancy

- Cleft lip with or without cleft palate (3 per cent)
- Skeletal abnormalities (1.9 per cent)
- Heart lesions (1.4 per cent)
- Nervous system defects (1.2 per cent)
- Alimentary system lesions (1.1 per cent)
- Face and ear abnormalities (1 per cent)
- Mental retardation (0.7 per cent)
- Lesions in the genitourinary system (0.6 per cent)

PARKINSON'S DISEASE

Parkinsonism, a condition affecting 1 in 1000 of the population, is the second commonest chronic disabling neurological disorder, vascular disease being the commonest. It can result from several spontaneously occurring and toxin-induced lesions of the nigrostriatal pathway. Parkinson's disease is a condition of unknown cause with degeneration of dopaminergic fibres in the nigrostriatal tracts plus appearances in the brain indistinguishable from Alzheimer's disease (senile plaques, neurofibrillary tangles and granulovacuolar degeneration). Neurological features are bradykinesia, rigidity and tremor. In addition, psychological problems often accompany these: depression; reduction in sexual performance; and periods of insomnia and nocturnal confusion associated with nightmares and hallucinations. The mental picture may thus be a constant one of moderate or severe depression or a fluctuating course of psychotic illness. Dementia frequently develops.

Treatment has greatly improved the quality and length of survival in these patients, but the long-term consequences of the disease are still not understood.

Anticholinergic drugs in Parkinson's disease

The anticholinergic drugs (such as benzhexol and benztropine) were the main type of treatment before the introduction of levodopa. They are still used in those patients who cannot tolerate adequate doses of levodopa, and are very effective in the early prodromal phase of the disease which presents as muscle pains most severe at night. At this stage there is no motor disorder, but anticholinergics can abolish the pain, although they can produce acute excited and confusional states particularly in the elderly. In view of the loss of cholinergic fibres in Alzheimer's disease, it is perhaps not surprising that anticholinergic drugs sometimes produce such problems in these patients.

Levodopa

The use of levodopa (with a decarboxylase inhibitor such as benserazide or carbidopa) is the drug of choice in established disease. The bradykinesia and rigidity are particularly improved and the total disability is greatly reduced in 70 per cent of patients. Treatment failures are due to unacceptable toxicity (or to incorrect diagnosis). The mental state can be greatly improved in patients on levodopa and depression may be abolished.

G. M. Stern and his colleagues in University College Hospital, London, followed 178 patients treated this way for over 6 years[36]. Dystonic reactions commonly complicated prolonged treatment with levodopa, but psychiatric complications were the most serious toxic effects and most frequently determined reduction in drug dose or even removal from treatment. The commonest serious psychiatric toxic effects were toxic confusional states, visual hallucinations and paranoid psychoses; 22 per cent of patients were depressed before the disease started and levodopa had no beneficial effect on this form of depression. After six years of treatment 32 per cent of patients had dementia, and cortical atrophy and ventricular dilatation were common.

It is not known if levodopa and anticholinergic drugs accelerated this degenerative process. Perhaps in the face of such uncertainty, even though levodopa remains the drug of first choice in Parkinson's disease, the maximum tolerated doses should not be used for long periods, but an alternative regime as suggested by Stern should be considered. This consists of using bromocriptine, an alternative dopamine agonist, combined with low doses of levodopa.

Alternative treatments include drugs which increase dopamine release, such as amantadine and selegiline, a selective monoamine oxidase B inhibitor (see table below). Both types of drug can produce mental changes – in particular, excitement and confusion.

The two forms of the enzyme monoamine oxidase

MAO-A	MAO-B
● Inhibited by: nialamide, iproniazid, phenelzine	● Inhibited by: selegiline
● Destroys: tyramine, hypertensive amines	● Does not destroy: tyramine, hypertensive amines
● Use of inhibitors: depression, phobic anxiety	● Use of inhibitors: Parkinson's disease (used with levodopa plus a decarboxylase inhibitor)
● When inhibited: hypertensive reactions with foods, e.g. cheese (tyramine), amphetamine, levodopa, ephedrine	● When inhibited: *no* hypertensive reactions with foods, amphetamine, levodopa, ephedrine

POSTCONCUSSIONAL SYNDROME

Distressing neurological and psychological symptoms are common sequelae of closed head injury. There is much controversy as to whether these are the result of organic brain damage or whether the symptoms are mostly of psychogenic origin. There is significant physical damage to the brain after even minor head injury. After a blow of sufficient severity to cause loss or other alteration in consciousness, lesions can be found in the medullary pontine nuclei and white matter.

Neurological disorders

Injuries to the head are now one of the commonest causes of neurological disorders. These are mainly a result of road traffic trauma, but falls and industrial accidents contribute as well. As the use of motor vehicles continues to rise, the number of people with head injuries also increases.

The spectrum of sequelae is broad. The milder and less tangible symptoms, which are not accompanied by physical signs, are headache, giddiness, irritability, depression, anxiety, poor concentration, faulty memory, sensitivity to alcohol, loss of libido and impotence. In some individuals these appear to represent a psychological disturbance, which may be associated with claims for compensation. However, the fortuitous finding by a young man that he can no longer tolerate alcohol, for example, does suggest an organic lesion. A proportion of patients with minor symptoms do have objective evidence of brain damage: vestibular function, cerebral circulation, and blood–brain barrier permeability may be found to be abnormal.

Organic injury

Severe injury which produces loss of consciousness, temporary respiratory arrest, fall or rise in blood pressure, loss of eye reflexes and mass contraction of limbs all indicate organic injury. Within a few hours headache or change in consciousness may be due to delayed cerebral oedema, haemorrhage or fractures of bone.

Even though patients with high motivation to return to work do so more quickly than some unskilled workers, symptoms may be present in the former group eighteen months after the injury. The delayed signs and symptoms which suggest organic damage are: occipital and frontal headaches which are aggravated by lying down, bending forwards, raising intrathoracic and intra-abdominal pressure; intellectual and social deterioration; disorders of memory; short bouts of vertigo; fits. These may not appear until one to two years after the injury.

Non-organic injury

By contrast, patients who are obviously anxious, depressed or involved in claims for compensation may have symptoms which suggest a non-organic basis. These include pains all over the head, or like a steel band, or pressure. The pain is described as very severe, like a needle, terrible and constant, and may not respond to analgesics in the expected way. If relief is afforded by drugs it comes on in two or three minutes and lasts less than half an hour. The pain may make the patient cry out, sigh or groan and there may be spasm of the frontalis or occipital muscles.

Chronic symptoms of such a neurotic nature are difficult to treat, although it may be possible to discuss the generation of the clinical picture by feelings of anxiety and tension. Drug therapy – in particular long-term administration of anxiolytics and hypnotics – may well aggravate the problem.

TICS

A tic is a purposeless, repetitive movement usually brief and jerky in nature. A spasm is an involuntary movement which is either sustained or clonic in nature. There is an overlap in the two conditions, and frequently the term tic is used to describe both.

Tics develop in over 10 per cent of children, and boys are affected much more frequently than girls. Tic movements most frequently involve the head or neck, and become increasingly uncommon towards the periphery of the body. Common forms are blinking, grimacing and lip and mouth movements. They are made worse when the patient is upset or is conscious of being observed and they disappear during sleep.

The commonest age of onset is seven years. The majority greatly improve or disappear within five years of onset. Tics which persist appear to be associated with unsympathetic and bullying reactions in parents, teachers and classmates.

Gilles de la Tourette syndrome

An unusual form of the condition is the Gilles de la Tourette syndrome. In this the onset may be delayed until the early teens and is characterized by the appearance of multiple tics and include those of speech, the latter taking the form of repetitive obscene phrases or echolalia. The syndrome tends to persist although there may be temporary remissions. Psychotic illness is not associated with it.

Management of tics

The management of simple tics should involve as little drama as possible. There should be no suggestion to the child that he is doing something wrong or peculiar. Parental pressures in relation to the tic and in other directions (such as demanding improved performance at school) should be removed immediately, if necessary by firm, directive instruction to the parents; 90 per cent of tics will cease on their own particularly if emotional tensions are reduced. Ridicule will cause them to persist.

In unusual cases when the tic is severe, relaxation techniques, meditation and hypnosis should be used before drug treatment is considered. In the most severely affected children who have failed to respond to other treatment, neuroleptic treatment is used. Haloperidol is most widely used, and may be successful, but acute dystonic reactions, parkinsonism and tardive dyskinesias can complicate prolonged treatment with neuroleptics. Because of this the smallest effective doses should be used for the shortest possible time.

ENDOCRINE DISORDERS

Thyroid disease

Disease of the thyroid gland is common. The prevalence is in excess of 3 per 10,000 adults per year, the sex ratio being 5:1, with a preponderance of women. Although hypothyroidism may present as mental slowing and hyperthyroidism as anxiety and agitation, the paradox of thyroid disease is that hypothyroidism often produces anxiety and hyperthyroidism may present as depression. One form of myxoedema madness is paranoia and this may accompany episodes of confusion in a patient with progressive dementia. The mental slowing of myxoedema can precede other clinical changes by several years. Treatment with thyroxine usually abolishes the psychiatric disturbances.

Cushing's syndrome

Adrenal insufficiency characteristically can present with the features of mild chronic dementia plus depressive features. Less frequently irritability, confusion and delusions have been observed. In Cushing's syndrome alterations in mood are common, usually consisting of irritability and easily provoked crying. Some patients are depressed and this has led to suicide. Manic behaviour is also described in Cushing's syndrome.

When the condition is due to disease of the adrenal cortex, surgical treatment usually abolishes the psychiatric symptoms. When the syndrome arises due to drug therapy, then mental illness may become an indication to withdraw the steroid.

Other syndromes

Hypopituitarism and hypocalcaemia may initially present as anxiety. Hyperparathyroidism with hypercalcaemia may produce feelings of weakness, fatiguability, anorexia, lack of energy, mood lability and depression.

Hypoglycaemia, if severe, can cause rapid unconsciousness, fits or death. If the patient recovers there may be evidence of residual brain damage. More mild and prolonged hypoglycaemia may be associated with confusion, hallucinations, aimless hyperactivity, anxiety, sweating and tremor. Acute hypoglycaemia is a medical emergency and should be terminated as soon as possible by intravenous injection of glucose as a 50 per cent solution.

PSYCHOTROPIC DRUGS IN PAINFUL CONDITIONS

The sensation of pain has complex associations with the emotions. The pain threshold varies according to the mood of the patient and the setting of the pain: fear, loneliness, depression and anxiety all lower the threshold, while feelings of optimism, interest in the environment and confidence about the successful outcome of treatment raise the pain threshold. Pain itself produces anxiety and depression and the recent experience of pain is itself hyperalgesic.

A common problem in rheumatoid arthritis is depression, partly related to the increasing dependence of the patient on others. Sometimes such depression may respond to antidepressive therapy, although more usually a good response to anti-inflammatory drugs and physiotherapy is more valuable.

Some mental illness can present with pain as the main clinical feature. For instance, atypical facial pain may not respond to analgesics but reveal its depressive nature by being alleviated by antidepressants. Some forms of atypical facial pain prove particularly refractory to treatment, and only respond to ECT or to combined drug therapy with an antidepressant and a neuroleptic.

Migraine can be triggered by depressive illness or by anxiety (see Chapter 12). In both circumstances antidepressant drugs may reduce the frequency of attacks or even abolish them. Long-term treatment with anxiolytics is not recommended. Similarly, migrainous neuralgia can respond to antidepressants in certain patients.

Analgesic use in terminal disease

In advanced malignant disease, pain may be due to invasion of tissue with direct involvement of nerve terminals. However, other causes are common.

Causes of pain in advanced malignant disease

- Invasion of tissue
- Constipation and haemorrhoids
- Musculoskeletal pain
- Bedsores
- Infection
- Venous thrombosis
- Pulmonary embolus

The most important aggravating factors are anxiety, fear and depression. The correct use of analgesics will do much to alleviate the psychological distress of terminal illness. The first analgesics to be used in such an illness are not necessarily the most powerful available. Paracetamol or an NSAID may prove to be successful. Metastases in bone produce erosion, vasodilatation and hence pain partly because of release of a prostaglandin (PGE). Aspirin and similar drugs act by blocking the synthesis of PGE and may in this way alleviate the pain of bony metastases.

Specific drug treatment Chronic cancer pain can usually only be controlled with narcotic analgesics. A sequence of increasing effectiveness is codeine, dihydrocodeine, Diconal (a mixture of dipipanone with cyclizine), and phenazocine. The most potent group includes morphine, diamorphine, methadone, levallorphan and buprenorphine. These drugs have to be given in sufficient doses to relieve the pain and at intervals such that the pain does not reappear before the next dose. PRN or 'when required' prescribing is wrong in painful malignant disease. Where possible these drugs are given orally; 80 per cent of patients with painful terminal disease never need more than 20 mg of diamorphine orally (the range of oral doses of diamorphine is 2.5–90 mg, equivalent to injections of 1–30 mg).

Psychological aspects of terminal pain

The peculiar features of terminal pain are that it is meaningless, tends to get worse and it is impossible to predict when it will end. These aspects of the physical distress are most demoralizing psychologically. However, they underline how vital it is for the physician to pay great attention to every detail of treatment and abolish the pain as completely and continuously as possible. Fears in relation to possible addiction are groundless. Patients who demand frequent injections and are anxious about their timing have been maintained on inadequate doses of analgesic. The appropriate doses for a patient will abolish the fear and memory of the pain. Psychological dependence is a desire to take a drug repeatedly in order to experience its psychological effects. This does not develop when narcotic analgesics are used as described above for pain control. Physical dependence does develop, and is common when narcotics have been used for three weeks or more. Patients whose painful condition abates can be gradually withdrawn from narcotic analgesics with no residual dependence.

Adding neuroleptics

The addition of a neuroleptic such as chlorpromazine can have several uses. The nausea and vomiting induced by the narcotic analgesic is suppressed and its action in reducing the fear and anxiety produced by pain is potentiated. When nausea due to the illness itself is severe, trifluoperazine or perphenazine may prove to have a more powerful antiemetic action.

At St Christopher's Hospice, London, methotrimeprazine is used when fear or dread accompanies nausea and pain. Chlorpromazine or promazine are also found to be effective in the control of delirium, confusion and other psychotic manifestations. Narcotic–neuroleptic combinations initially produce much sleepiness, but this does not usually persist beyond two or three days. Oral analgesic–neuroleptic mixtures do not usually produce respiratory depression unless large doses are used. The doses of some of the phenothiazines used in St Christopher's Hospice are as follows:

- Prochlorperazine:
  5 mg, 4–8-hourly orally
  12.5 mg, 8-hourly by injection
  25 mg, 8-hourly by suppository
- Chlorpromazine:
  12.5–25 mg, 4-hourly orally
  25 mg, 4–8-hourly by injection
  100 mg, 8-hourly by suppository

Other agents

Metoclopramide is useful for centrally induced vomiting and nausea due to delayed gastric emptying. It has no sedative action, and little or no antipsychotic activity. Cyclizine is an alternative antiemetic used with narcotic analgesics. Domperidone is similar to metoclopramide, but is less likely to produce dystonic reactions.

Antidepressants and anxiolytics About one-quarter of terminally ill patients at St Christopher's Hospice are also prescribed a tricyclic antidepressant or benzodiazepine. As in other areas of medicine, the tricyclics can be used for long periods (up to six months) if there is an accompanying depressive illness, but the benzodiazepines are only used for short periods of severe anxiety.

Cocaine is used in some centres to potentiate the analgesic effect of narcotic analgesics and reduce their sedative actions. Temporary benefit is experienced by some patients but the improvement is not usually maintained.

Steroids Pain due to nerve compression or raised intracranial pressure may be relieved by steroids. The glucocorticoid most commonly used for this is dexamethasone in an initial dose of 16 mg (or more) daily. Steroids are also effective in some patients with anorexia, depression and lethargy. A suitable regime for this is prednisolone 15 mg daily.

PRACTICAL POINTS

- It is possible that there is a psychological component in the causation of all physical illnesses. Significant life events appear to act as triggers for the appearance of physical illness.
- In hyperventilation the best treatments are muscle relaxation techniques and breathing exercises.
- Psychological factors play a considerable part in gastrointestinal disorders.
- Asthma should be treated with beta-agonists and steroids, but *never* with anxiolytics.
- Phenytoin is the most useful anticonvulsant in the treatment of major epilepsy, but carbamazepine, sodium valproate, phenobarbitone and primidone are also effective.
- Most sufferers from Parkinson's disease benefit from treatment by levodopa, but serious psychiatric complications can occur.
- Injuries to the head are one of the commonest causes of neurological disorders.
- Haloperidol is the most widely used drug in the treatment of tics, but drugs are rarely required.
- In terminal disease it is vital for the physician to pay great attention to every detail of treatment and abolish the pain as completely and continuously as possible.

12
Migraine and other types of headache

BACKGROUND

Migraine appears to be a vascular disorder, characterized by excessive reactivity of arteries in the skull and surface of the brain. In some instances, chemical trigger factors, such as foodstuffs, are identified. There are, however, patients in whom anxiety or depression, or the relief from a worry can trigger attacks of migraine.

The majority of causes of headache are benign; nevertheless a large proportion of patients with organic disease of the brain, eyes, temporomandibular joint, sinuses, cervical spine and cranial blood vessels experience pain. Intracranial tumours and aneurysms can produce a clinical picture similar to migraine or cluster headache.

MIGRAINE

Twenty per cent of men and 30 per cent of women are thought to suffer from migraine. Several types of migraine are described. In some instances the management differs according to the type of migraine experienced. In classical migraine the headache is preceded or accompanied by sensory or motor phenomena, which most commonly consist of disturbances in a visual field. However, the aura may take the form of paraesthesia, speech disturbances or paralysis.

The headache itself typically is unilateral, spreading from the region of the upper eyelid over the top of the head, sometimes as far as the occiput. The headache may be severe and throbbing and can be accompanied by nausea and vomiting. Some patients find that attacks can only be terminated by sleep. The pain may last from half an hour to more than a day. Some sufferers may experience one or two attacks a year, while others may have several attacks each week.

The course of the condition is very variable. In some people the attacks begin in childhood and continue throughout life. In others they may only appear in old age, or during the course of two or three years following the menopause, or may only be experienced while taking the contraceptive pill.

DRUGS USED IN AN ACUTE ATTACK OF MIGRAINE

- Minor analgesics
- Anxiolytics
- Antiemetics
- Ergotamine

Minor analgesics

The majority of patients suffering from the headache of acute migraine can be helped with aspirin (900 mg) or paracetamol (1 g). In some patients the nausea of the migraine attack is worsened by aspirin. Narcotic analgesics are contraindicated but some neurologists treat their own migraine with codeine.

Anxiolytics

Many patients retire to bed during an attack. Relaxation and sleep are facilitated by prescribing a benzodiazepine such as diazepam (5 mg). However, sedatives make the ambulant patient feel worse.

Antiemetics

Migraine frequently provokes nausea and vomiting. Even when these are not features of an attack, gastric emptying is delayed and the absorption of analgesics is impaired. In both these circumstances metoclopramide can be very helpful. It inhibits the chemoreceptor trigger zone in the brain (and thus has a central antiemetic action) and also enhances gastric emptying, pyloric opening and peristalsis in the small intestine. A dose of 10 mg given fifteen minutes before administration of an analgesic will accelerate the absorption of the latter. If vomiting is severe, intramuscular metoclopramide (10 mg/2 ml) or prochlorperazine suppositories (25 mg) may be required. Paramax is a combined preparation, each tablet or sachet containing 500 mg of paracetamol with 5 mg of metoclopramide. Some patients respond to two of these at the onset of an attack. Domperidone has a similar peripheral action to metoclopramide but less enters the brain to produce extrapyramidal toxicity.

Ergotamine tartrate

This is used if the above measures alone are not successful. The two important points concerning this drug are:

1. To give it as early as possible in the acute attack (although the aura may be aggravated by ergotamine).
2. To administer the correct dose.

Excessive doses can produce nausea, vomiting and headache, which might be misinterpreted by the patient as indications for more ergotamine; this can have disastrous results.

Dose and effects The usual appropriate oral adult dose of ergotamine tartrate is 1 mg per attack; 0.25 mg is the intramuscular dose of dihydroergotamine. The following may be used in an acute migraine attack:

Ergotamine preparations

Preparation	Ergotamine content	Administration	Dose per attack
Lingraine (UK)	2 mg/tablet	Sublingually	½ tablet (1 tablet may be excessive)
Lingraine (Austr)	1 mg/tablet	Sublingually	1 tablet
Medihaler Ergotamine (UK)	0.36 mg/puff	By inhalation	2 puffs
Medihaler Ergotamine (Austr)	0.45 mg/puff	By inhalation	2 puffs
Cafergot	1 mg ergotamine plus 100 mg caffeine/tablet	Orally	1 tablet
Cafergot Suppository (UK) Cafergot PB Suppository (Austr)	2 mg and other agents/ suppository	Per rectum	½ suppository
Migril (UK) Migral (Austr)	2 mg ergotamine plus 50 mg cyclizine plus 100 mg caffeine/tablet	Orally	½ tablet (1 tablet may be excessive)

The injection form of ergotamine has been withdrawn but injected dihydroergotamine is less toxic. Dihydergot is also available as 1 mg tablets and as an oral liquid (2 mg/ml).

Toxic effects of ergotamine

- Anorexia, nausea, vomiting
- Cold extremities, Raynaud's phenomenon, claudication, gangrene, headache
- Mental changes, confusion

Case history: atypical migraine

A female tap dancer aged forty-two started to experience attacks of aching pain and lachrymation in the right eye at about the time of menstruation. The pain lasted about a day and was accompanied by blockage of the right nostril. The attacks were not affected by aspirin, paracetamol or ibuprofen. However, when ergotamine tartrate (1 puff of a Medihaler) was used, the attacks were stopped within ten minutes. Presumably these episodes were atypical migraine, with features of both cluster headache and migrainous neuralgia.

MIGRAINE PROPHYLAXIS

Migraine may become more troublesome or even appear for the first time during periods of distress, anxiety or depression. If these can be helped then the frequency of attacks may be reduced.

Similarly, precipitating factors such as missed meals, chocolate, alcohol, cheese or fruit should be identified and avoided. If oral contraceptives provoke migraine or substantially aggravate it then this method of contraception must be withdrawn.

If more than two attacks occur in a month, prophylactic drugs may be indicated. These should be reviewed every four to six months and stopped as soon as feasible.

Prophylactic agents for migraine

- Antidepressants
- Anticonvulsants
- Beta-blockers
- Pizotifen
- Clonidine
- Dihydroergotamine
- Methysergide
- Lithium

Antidepressants

Although the use of antidepressants (such as amitriptyline or phenelzine) may be successful in the treatment of depressed individuals presenting with classical migraine or atypical facial pain, the long-term use of anxiolytics cannot be justified even in patients with overt anxiety neurosis associated with migraine. Drugs such as diazepam lose their effectiveness after chronic use for two or three weeks and dependence can develop.

Anticonvulsants

These are an effective prophylactic in a small proportion of migraine sufferers. Phenytoin (starting dose 200 mg at night) or carbamazepine (100 mg 12-hourly) are used.

Beta-blockers

Beta-blockers such as propranolol and atenolol are useful in some patients, but the dose has to be adjusted to the individual needs of the patient. There is much variation in the optimal dose of propranolol but atenolol is usually effective at 100 mg daily.

Pizotifen

This is a 5-HT receptor blocker. Some patients respond well on doses of 5 mg 8–12-hourly. Pizotifen is sedating and stimulates the appetite, so weight gain may become a problem.

Clonidine

This agent in low doses (25–50 μg 8–12-hourly) is useful in classical migraine, particularly if there is a dietary precipitating factor. But even in these low doses drowsiness, dry mouth and depression can occur.

Dihydroergotamine

This is used by some physicians as a prophylactic for short periods. However, only during severe bouts of cluster headache or migrainous neuralgia is ergotamine considered as a prophylactic agent. The daily dose is 1–2 mg, but treatment should be supervised by an expert in this field.

Methysergide

This powerful 5-HT antagonist and vasoconstrictor is a dangerous drug and only rarely used. The dose is 1–2 mg 8-hourly. The most serious toxic effects develop after seven months' treatment and because of this the maximum course of treatment is six months.

Toxic effects of methysergide

- Nausea, vomiting, diarrhoea, abdominal pain
- Dysphoria, dissociation, hyperaesthesia
- Weight gain, oedema
- Angina, intermittent claudication, hypertension
- Retroperitoneal fibrosis, mediastinal fibrosis

Lithium

Lithium carbonate given in doses to maintain plasma levels at 0.6–1 mEq/l may be an effective prophylactic in cluster headache.

HEADACHE

Tension headache

The commonest type of headache is tension headache (psychogenic, anxiety, depressive or muscle contraction headache). This affects over three-quarters of the population. In some patients reassurance and sympathy may be the only therapy needed once the benign nature of the condition has been established. Relaxation techniques, perhaps involving biofeedback, can be very effective if the patient is able to learn these.

In the management of an acute attack some physicians prescribe analgesics such as aspirin or paracetamol, but there is no convincing evidence that these produce results better than a placebo (which admittedly may be considerable). There is also no clear reason why analgesics should be effective in tension headache. As well as relaxation and meditation techniques, active exercise regimes can also be helpful. In the unusual instances when tension headaches are part of a serious psychological disturbance appropriate psychotherapy and drug therapy may be required. In general, the long-term use of anxiolytic agents is not recommended.

Cluster headache

Cluster headache (migrainous neuralgia; Horton's histamine cephalalgia) is much less common than tension headache and probably occurs in 0.5–1 per cent of the population. The majority of patients are men. The pain is usually distressing and often has a burning quality. It is usually accompanied by anxiety and there is ipsilateral blockage of the nose, nasal discharge and conjunctival redness. The headaches may come on regularly for many years but may occur frequently during a period of a month or more. Each attack typically lasts one to three hours.

Treatment Cluster headaches commonly respond to simple analgesics or, if necessary, to oral ergotamine. Severe headaches may require injections of ergotamine or ergotamine inhalations via an aerosol. The most severe and refractory forms of the condition may respond to chlorpromazine, a drug that can be used for both the acute attack and for prophylaxis. As mentioned previously in this chapter lithium carbonate may be effective in the prophylaxis of cluster headache.

Trigeminal neuralgia

Trigeminal neuralgia characteristically presents as brief attacks of severe lancinating pain provoked by stimulation of trigger points. The pain spreads within one division of the sensory distribution of the trigeminal nerve.

Treatment The response to carbamazepine is often so satisfactory that such an improvement confirms the original diagnosis. The starting dose is 50–100 mg two or three times daily, increasing until improvement results or toxicity develops. The usual dose-limiting toxicity is fatigue, drowsiness, weakness, giddiness and unsteadiness of gait.

Patients intolerant to carbamazepine may respond to phenytoin (usually 100–400 mg given once daily), and the addition of chlorpromazine or an antidepressant may improve the response to these drugs.

Patients who fail to respond to drug therapy may have to be referred for specialist treatment such as peripheral neurectomy, trigeminal ganglion injection, microvascular decompression or percutaneous radio-frequency trigeminal neurolysis.

PRACTICAL POINTS

- Carbamazepine is the drug of choice in the treatment of trigeminal neuralgia.
- Migraine attacks can be terminated in 75 per cent of patients with aspirin (900 mg) or paracetamol (1 g).
- If nausea is present, metoclopramide 10 mg can be taken fifteen minutes before these analgesics.
- If analgesics fail, ergotamine tartrate can be used, the dose being 1 mg orally (higher doses may produce nausea and headache).
- Prophylactic therapy (e.g. pizotifen or beta-blockers) is only used if more than two attacks occur each month.
- The long-term use of anxiolytic agents is not recommended in tension headache, but lithium carbonate may be effective in the prophylaxis of cluster headache.

13
Essentials of pharmacokinetics

BACKGROUND

Pharmacokinetics has been defined as dealing with the mathematical description of biological processes which affect drugs and those which are affected *by* drugs. These processes include drug absorption, distribution, metabolism and elimination. In addition to investigation of these individual areas, pharmacokinetics is useful to practitioners for the assessment of the relationship of the dose administered to the plasma drug concentration; it may also sometimes be of value to predict the clinical effects of a drug. This concluding chapter summarizes basic pharmacokinetic concepts.

Much of the pharmacokinetic literature is concerned with the analysis of blood or plasma concentration/time curves and this forms a convenient place to start this summary.

ANALYSIS OF BLOOD AND PLASMA

If a single dose of a drug is injected as a bolus into the circulation, a peak plasma level is, to all intents, immediately obtained and then subsides. This fall is due to a combination of drug redistribution (out of the vascular system into the tissues) and drug elimination by metabolism and/or excretion. A very common pattern of behaviour resembles the decay of a radioactive isotope or of an electrical charge on a condenser and is shown in Figure 9.

As can be seen, the rate of fall in plasma concentration is not constant with time but falls more slowly as the drug level decreases. Just like radioactive decay the process is described by an exponential equation

$$C_t = C_0 e^{-kt} \qquad (1)$$

where C_t is the concentration at time t; C_0 is the initial plasma concentration; k is first-order rate constant and expresses the extent to which the drug is eliminated in unit time. For example, if $k = 0.5\ h^{-1}$ then half of the substance is removed in 1 hour. Thus a value of $0.25\ h^{-1}$ represents slower elimination than 0.5 and a value of 1 implies a more rapid elimination.

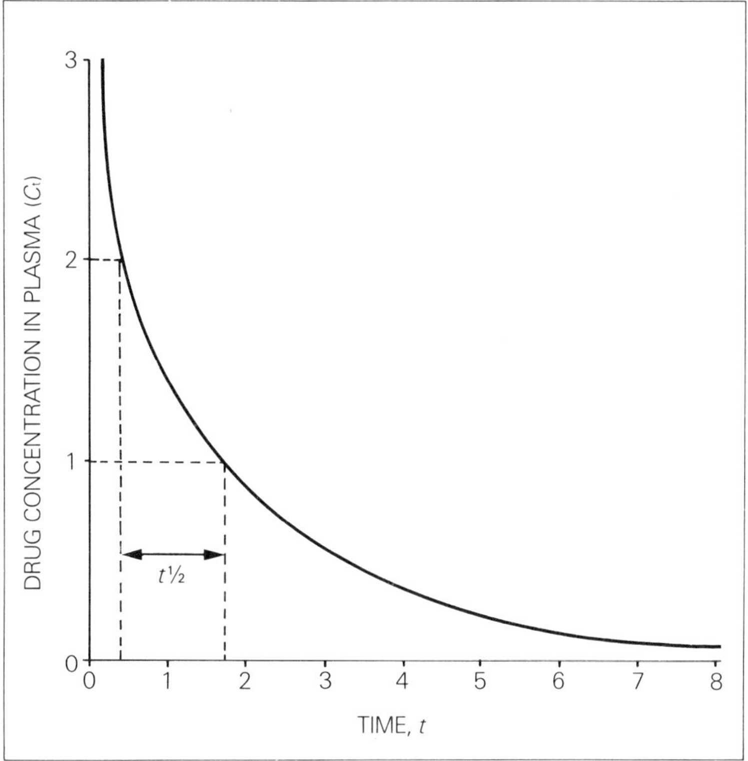

Figure 9 Exponential fall in plasma drug concentration when plotted on linear scales; ($t_{1/2}$ = half time of elimination and is constant for first-order kinetics).

e is the base of natural logarithms and so

$$ln\ C_t = ln\ C_o - kt \tag{2}$$

and because 2.303 log a = $ln\ a$ equation (1) may also be written

$$\log C_t = \log C_o \frac{-kt}{2.303} \tag{3}$$

It is often useful therefore to use a semilog plot to express the decline of plasma concentrations (Figure 10) since this converts the curve of Figure 9 to a straight line, which is mathematically more tractable.

On log-linear plots k is given by slope × 2.303 as implied by equation (3). Equations (1) or (3) may also be used to predict the fall in plasma concentration with time, since given any point on the curve (= C_t) the concentration after a time interval t has elapsed may be calculated if k is known.

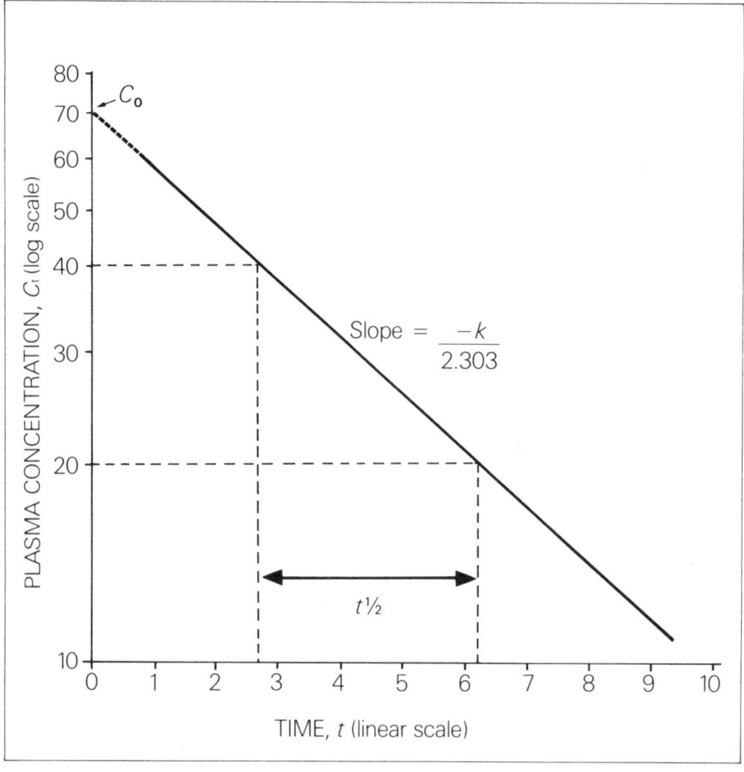

Figure 10 Plotting an exponential decline in plasma concentration on log-linear scales gives a straight line; $t_{½}$ is again constant.

Half-life

The half-life of a drug ($t_{½}$) is the time required for the plasma drug concentration to fall by one half. Substitution in equation (1) gives

$$\frac{C_o}{2} = C_o\, e^{-kt_{½}} \tag{4}$$

Dividing by C_o yields $\frac{1}{2} = e^{-kt_{½}}$, which put into natural logarithms is

$$ln\,\frac{1}{2} = -kt_{½}$$

Multiplying by -1 gives

$$-ln\,\frac{1}{2} = kt_{½}$$

Since $\quad -ln\frac{1}{2} = 0.693$

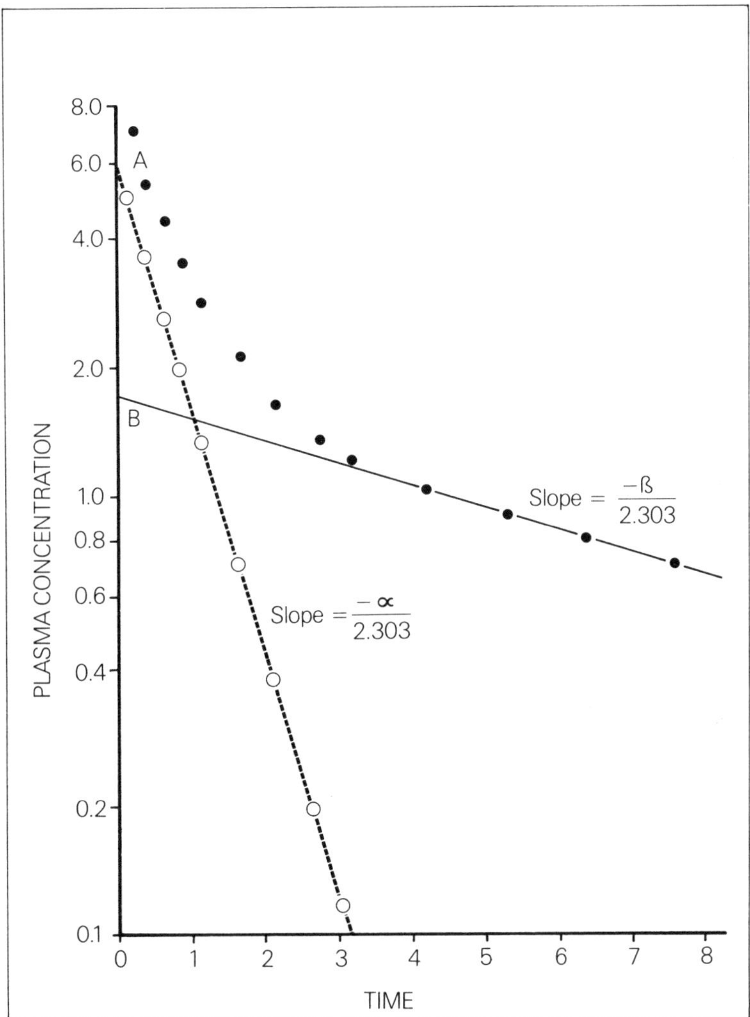

Figure 11 Plasma concentration/time curve for a drug conferring the characteristics of a two-compartment system on the body. The second (β) phase of the curve has a slope of $\frac{-\beta}{2.303}$ and back extrapolation (—) gives B, the ordinate intercept. Subtraction of concentrations predicted by this line at times corresponding to data points yields points (o-----o) which lie on a straight line with ordinate intercept A and slope $\frac{-\alpha}{2.303}$.

we have

$$t_{1/2} = \frac{0.693}{k} \tag{5}$$

In practice $t_{1/2}$ is usually found from the log-linear plot of drug concentration; time and k can be calculated from equation (5).

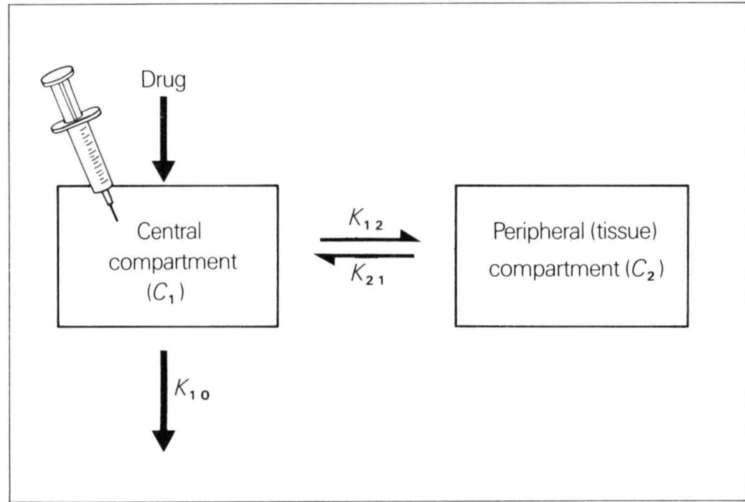

Figure 12 The two-compartment pharmacokinetic model.

Multicompartment models

So far we have made the assumption that the body may be simply represented mathematically as a homogeneous, well-stirred compartment in which the drug is distributed instantaneously. In practice this is often too naive, and instead of a straight line on the log-linear plot an inflected line with more than one slope is found (Figure 11).

Here the initial (or α) phase corresponds to a period during which the drug is mainly distributing in the body (although some elimination is occurring) and the secondary (or β) phase represents mainly elimination (with some redistribution). Conceptually this may be considered as taking place in a two-compartment system as shown in Figure 12.

These compartments have no physiological or anatomical reality but it is assumed that sampling (i.e. from the blood) takes place from the central compartment. The brain may be in either compartment and such models are not useful for the estimation of actual tissue levels of a drug. As might be expected from equation (1) this two-compartment system is described by a double exponential equation:

$$C_t = Ae^{-\alpha t} + Be^{-\beta t} \tag{6}$$

α is the rate constant for the first phase and β is the rate constant for the second phase of the curve. The latter is often called the beta phase; when a half-life is quoted without qualification it is assumed that $t_{1/2}$ $\left(= \frac{0.693}{\beta}\right)$ is meant. During the beta phase the drug levels in both compartments decline in parallel. The zero time intercept obtained by extrapolation of the terminal linear beta-phase to $t=0$ is B. A may be obtained by firstly subtracting the values for C_t on this line from the plasma concentration/time curve

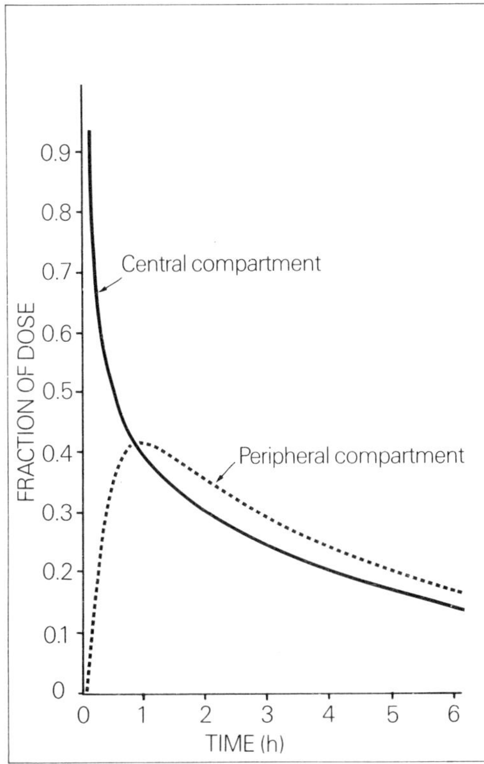

Figure 13 Semilog plot of concentrations in blood (compartment 1) and tissue (compartment 2) following an intravenous dose of drug. Loss of drug from blood and tissues is represented by parallel lines during the beta phase.

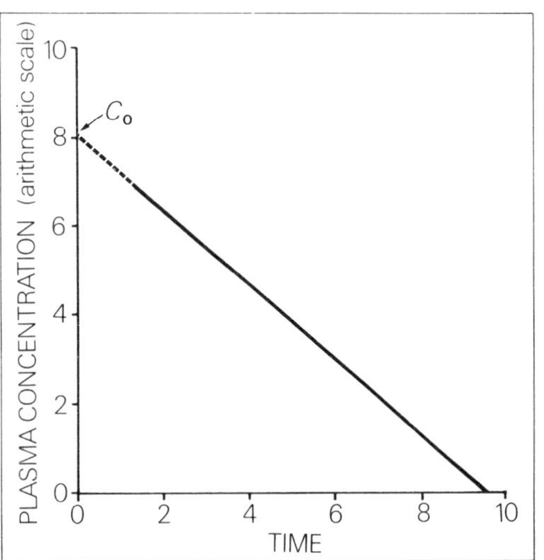

Figure 14 Decline of plasma drug concentration obeying zero-order kinetics yields a straight line on linear scales but $t_{1/2}$ is not constant and is longer at higher concentrations.

which yields a second straight line with a zero-time intercept A and slope = $-\alpha/2.303$ (Figure 13).

During the beta phase equilibration has been attained between plasma and tissues (Figure 14), but it should be realized that the tissue drug levels do not equal the plasma level but only parallel them. The value of plasma level monitoring of drugs is dependent upon this parallelism and assumes that the ratio of drug in plasma and tissue is relatively constant between different individuals. Therefore, blood samples for monitoring of drug levels must be taken during the beta phase.

In a similar way, if there are three linear segments to the log concentration/time plot the kinetics require a triexponential equation for the three compartments necessary to describe this behaviour.

The apparent volume of distribution

The apparent volume of distribution of a drug, which confers the properties of a single compartment system on the body, is easily understood and is calculated from

$$C_o = \frac{D}{V_d} \tag{7}$$

where D is the dose of drug administered and V_d is the apparent volume of distribution. Since D is the total amount of drug in the body at zero time, we can write more generally

$$X_t = C_t \, V_d \tag{8}$$

where X_t is the amount of drug in the body at any time t.

Equation (8) states that the apparent volume of distribution is the factor by which the plasma concentration must be multiplied to determine the amount of drug in the body. Like the compartmental concept it has no anatomical reality and is in this sense a mathematical fiction. Indeed, in the case of drugs which, like many psychotropics, are highly protein bound or lipid soluble the apparent volume of distribution can exceed the total volume of the body, sometimes severalfold. Nevertheless, if the apparent volume of distribution is around 0.7 l/kg bodyweight it is often assumed that the drug is distributed throughout the body water.

The concept of apparent volume of distribution becomes complicated when it is applied to multicompartment systems, and there is controversy about which is the most appropriate technique for its estimation. The two which are most commonly quoted are:

1. $V_{d\beta}$ (also called $V_{d(area)}$) which is the apparent volume of distribution in the beta phase.

$$V_{d\beta} = \frac{D}{\beta\,(AUC)} \tag{9}$$

where AUC is the area under the plasma concentration/time curve.

2. V_c is the volume of the central compartment

$$V_c = \frac{D}{A + B} \tag{10}$$

The analogy of equation (10) with equation (7) should be noted.

Many psychoactive drugs have large apparent volumes of distribution and are therefore present in very low concentrations in the blood after distribution. This requires that pharmacokinetic studies on these drugs depend on sensitive and specific assay methods. Such techniques include gas-liquid chromatography, mass spectrometry, high performance thin layer chromatography (TLC) and radioimmunoassay.

Total body clearance of a drug (Cl)

This may be defined as the fraction of the apparent volume of distribution cleared from the body in unit time. As an index of drug elimination it is more meaningful than the plasma half-life since it is derived from the sum of all the clearance mechanisms and unlike $t_{1/2}$ or k it is independent of the apparent volume of distribution.

By definition

$$Cl = k\, V_d \tag{11}$$

and from equation (5) we therefore have

$$t_{1/2} = \frac{0.693\, V_d}{Cl} \tag{12}$$

Also by definition

Total body clearance = renal clearance + hepatic clearance
+ clearance by other routes (usually minor)

The upper limit of total body clearance is the flow throughout all the organs of elimination (usually liver and kidneys) and is about 0.04 l/kg/min. It is calculated from

$$Cl = \frac{D}{AUC} \tag{13}$$

Compare with equation (9). A further advantage is that it is practically model-independent.

The renal clearance of a drug is given by

$$Cl_r = \frac{\text{Total urinary drug excretion}}{AUC} \tag{14}$$

and the concept can also be extended to biliary and salivary elimination.

Oral or intramuscular drug administration

This gives a plasma concentration/time curve which shows a rising phase and one or more phases of decline. Such behaviour can be described for a one-compartment model by:

$$C_t = \frac{F\, D\, k_a}{V_d(k_a - k)}\left(e^{-k(t-t')} - e^{-k_a(t-t')}\right) \tag{15}$$

where k_a is a constant analogous to k_e which describes the rate of absorption from the gut or intramuscular injection site and t' is the lag time or time before drug is detected in the plasma.

Bioavailability fraction F is the fraction of the dose D which is systemically absorbed and is called the bioavailability fraction. Drugs which are completely absorbed have $F = 1$, but incompletely absorbed drugs have $F < 1$. Those drugs which are metabolized by the liver or gut wall before entering the systemic circulation (first-pass metabolism) despite complete or near-complete absorption also have $F < 1$. Examples of drugs undergoing extensive first-pass metabolism include chlorpromazine, imipramine and nortriptyline.

More complex equations describe absorption into two-compartment systems from oral or intramuscular administration.

DOSE-DEPENDENT KINETICS

Thus far it has been assumed that all the pharmacokinetic processes considered can be expressed by first-order linear differential equations of the type

$$\frac{dC}{dt} = -kC \tag{16}$$

for which equation (1) is the integrated solution. Equation (16) shows that the decrease of plasma concentration with time is proportional to the plasma concentration (k is a proportionality constant). Some biological processes may, however, be capacity-limited because of saturation of an enzyme or transport process. When saturation occurs the rate of drug elimination (or transfer) is limited and is described by so-called zero-order kinetics which is expressed by equation (17) – analogous to equation (16).

$$\frac{dC}{dt} = -k \tag{17}$$

for which the integrated solution is equation (18) – analogous to equation (1).

$$C_t = C_o - kt \tag{18}$$

This is the equation of a straight line (Figure 15).

For such processes the $t_{½}$ becomes longer the higher the dose and the total body clearance is also dose-dependent.

First-order and zero-order kinetics may be regarded as two different ends of the spectrum of processes obeying Michaelis–Menten kinetics which is described by

$$\frac{dC}{dt} = -\frac{V_{max}C}{K_m + C} \tag{19}$$

where V_{max} is the maximum rate of the process and K_m is the drug concentration at which the rate of the process is equal to one-half of V_{max}. When $C >> K_m$ the process is effectively zero-order, while if $K_m >> C$ the process obeys first-order kinetics. A number of drugs demonstrate capacity-limited elimination in the dose ranges encountered

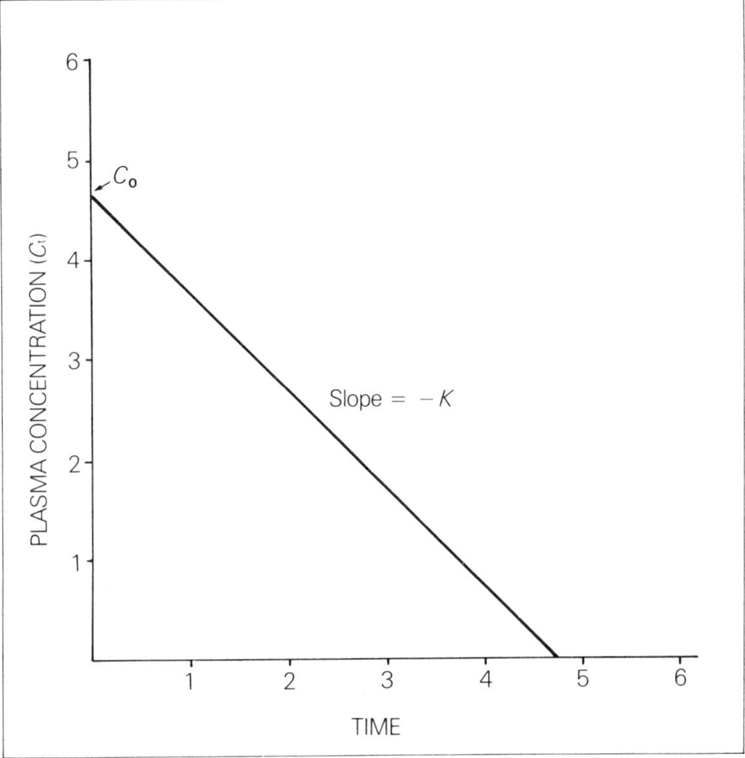

Figure 15 Fall in plasma concentration of a drug with time. Drug eliminated by zero-order kinetics. Initial concentration at time 0 is C_0.

in clinical practice, including ethanol, salicylate and phenytoin. The consequences of capacity-limited elimination include:

1. Variable $t_{1/2}$. This becomes longer with higher doses.
2. *AUC* is not proportional to dose (so called dose-dependence or non-linear behaviour).
3. Propensity to drug accumulation (and toxicity) when V_{max} is exceeded so that severalfold increases in steady-state levels may occur for small increases in dose.
4. Greater liability to drug–drug interactions due to competition for the rate limiting step.

MULTIPLE DOSING

In everyday practice multiple doses of drugs are usually administered repetitively at a constant dose interval (T). This results in the attainment of an average steady-state concentration C_{ss} which is expressed by the model-independent equation:

$$C_{ss} = \frac{F\ D}{V_d\ k\ T} \tag{20}$$

This may also be rearranged to give the dose interval or dose to achieve a given steady-state concentration.

The rate at which the equilibrium state is achieved (when amount of drug input during a dosage interval = amount of drug output during a dosage interval) is related to the $t_{1/2}$ of the drug and is independent of the dose. To a first approximation the steady state is reached after five half-lives have elapsed. The size of the dose, however, determines the level reached, hence the use of a larger loading dose to achieve the therapeutic range rapidly followed by a smaller maintenance dose. Such a manoeuvre is necessary when the long $t_{1/2}$ of the drug would require an impractically long period before the therapeutic range was attained by multiple dosing with the maintenance dose.

Assuming complete absorption, a drug will accumulate in the body if it is given at intervals less than 1.4 times its half-life. The accumulation ratio is the multiple by which the average amount of drug in the body at steady state following multiple dosing with fixed doses at a constant dosing interval T exceeds the amount administered in a single dose. This is given by:

$$R = \frac{1.4\ t_{1/2}}{T} \tag{21}$$

DRUG–PROTEIN BINDING

Drug binding to plasma and tissue protein has an important influence upon the distribution and pharmacological effects of a drug. Unbound drug is available to distribute into the tissue fluid and the apparent volume of distribution is related to plasma and tissue binding by

$$V_d = V_B + V_T\left(\frac{f_b}{f_t}\right) \tag{22}$$

where V_B and V_T are the actual volumes of water in blood and tissues respectively (that is, $V_B + V_T$ = total body water), and f_b and f_t are the fractions of free drug in blood and tissues respectively. Therefore changes in the unbound fraction of drug in plasma without commensurate changes in tissue binding alter the apparent volume of distribution.

Only free drug is available to interact with the tissue receptors to cross the blood–brain barrier and to undergo glomerular filtration. Penetration into saliva is often a passive process reflecting the amount of unbound drug in plasma so that salivary drug excretion can be used as a measure of the unbound drug fraction. Lithium, chlorpromazine and amitriptyline have been measured in saliva and, theoretically at least, saliva could be used to monitor drug therapy. Since the free fraction of drug is associated with drug activity it is conceivable that differences in drug response may be related to differences in the degree of protein binding between individuals. At present assay methods to establish whether this factor is of importance are too difficult to extend to routine clinical practice: salivary drug assay may eventually prove useful in this context.

Although plasma albumin is a major site of plasma drug binding, α_1-acid glycoprotein also avidly binds some basic drugs such as chlorpromazine, imipramine and propranolol. Since this protein is an acute phase reactant and its concentration is elevated three to four times when the erythrocyte sedimentation rate (ESR) rises in inflammatory disease, changes in protein binding of such drugs could be influenced by intercurrent disease. As yet the clinical relevance of this is not established.

CONCLUSION

To a certain extent the immediate clinical utility of pharmacokinetics to the practising doctor depends upon the relationship between the drug concentration in some easily sampled biological material and the drug effect. Psychiatry was one of the earliest disciplines to utilize drug level monitoring since Wuth in 1927 suggested the use of serum bromide concentrations as an adjunct to its national use as a sedative[37].

The criteria which make drug level monitoring a desirable procedure are:

1. The existence of a direct relationship between drug or metabolite concentration and pharmacological effect.
2. Drug effects that cannot readily be assessed by clinical observation.
3. The interindividual variability in plasma drug concentration which is wide and unpredictable.
4. The low therapeutic index of the drug.
5. The elimination of the drug by a saturable mechanism.
6. To determine patient compliance.
7. To investigate the effect of the patient's disease or other factors on drug kinetics.
8. The availability of a relatively inexpensive, rapid and accurate assay technique which gives reproducible results between different laboratories.

As in many other instances these criteria are only partially met by the drugs used in psychiatry.

As yet, unfortunately, pharmacokinetics is only minimally integrated with clinical practice.

PRACTICAL POINTS

- Pharmacokinetics is the study of all the factors which govern the concentration of drugs in body fluids. These factors are drug absorption, distribution, metabolism and excretion.
- Blood levels are only important in therapeutics if it can be shown that there is a relationship between drug concentration in the body and therapeutic actions of the drug.
- Most drugs are absorbed through the wall of the upper part of the small intestine. The drug then enters the portal blood and passes through the liver. If all the drug passes from the gut into the peripheral circulation then the bioavailability is said to be 1. If all the drug is not absorbed, or a fraction is destroyed on passage through the liver (first-pass metabolism), the bioavailability is a fraction representing the proportion of drug which enters the body.
- Elimination of drugs is by metabolic degradation or by excretion, or by a combination of these. The majority of drugs are eliminated by a first-order mechanism (i.e. an exponential loss – like decay of a radioactive substance). This means that the fall in blood concentration can be expressed in terms of half life ($t_{1/2}$). This is one of the pharmacokinetic constants which express how long a drug acts and how long (on repeated dosing) it takes to reach a steady state concentration in the blood.
- For those drugs whose elimination is mainly or entirely by hepatic metabolism, the $t_{1/2}$ can be shortened if another agent is given which stimulates the liver to destroy foreign compounds more rapidly. Such an agent is called an inducing agent and can greatly lessen the effectiveness of a drug.

Drug trade names

Please note

1. All trade names begin with a capital letter.
2. It should not be assumed that products containing the same active ingredient, but made by different manufacturers, are exactly equivalent in therapeutic effect. It is possible that such products contain differing amounts of active ingredient, or different non-active ingredients.
3. Single-ingredient products containing dihydrocodeine, contain much lower doses of dihydrocodeine in Australia than those in Britain. The Australian products are used as cough suppressants, whereas those in Britain are used as analgesics.
4. The Australian product containing sterculia (Normacol) is not indicated for use in the treatment of obesity.

Key
* – combination product
** – discontinued product

British generic name	British trade name	Australian trade name
amantadine	Symmetrel	Symmetrel; Antadine
amitriptyline	Tryptizol Saroten Elavil Domical	Tryptanol Elavil Saroten Laroxyl Amitrip
amyl nitrite	not available**	unbranded product only
amylobarbitone sodium	Sodium Amytal	Amytal Sodium Amylobeta Neur-Amyl Sodium

British generic name	British trade name	Australian trade name
atenolol	Tenormin	Tenormin
baclofen	Lioresal	Lioresal
benperidol	Anquil	not available
benserazide	Madopar*	Madopar*
benzhexol	Artane	Artane Anti-Spas
benztropine	Cogentin	Cogentin
betahistine	Serc	Serc
bethanidine	Esbatal	Esbatal
bromocriptine	Parlodel	Parlodel
buprenorphine	Temgesic	Temgesic
butriptyline	Evadyne	not available
carbamazepine	Tegretol	Tegretol Convuline
carbidopa	Sinemet*	Sinemet*
chloral hydrate	Noctec	Noctec
chlordiazepoxide	Librium Tropium	Librium
chlormethiazole	Heminevrin	Hemineurin
chlormezanone	Trancopal	not available
chlorpromazine	Largactil Chloractil	Largactil Protran Procalm Promacid
chlorprothixene	Taractan	not available
clobazam	Frisium	not available
clomipramine	Anafranil	Anafranil
clonazepam	Rivotril	Rivotril
clonidine	Dixarit	Dixarit
clopenthixol	Clopixol	not available
clopenthixol decanoate	Clopixol (injection)	not available
clorazepate	Tranxene	Tranxene
clothiapine	not available	not available
clozapine	not available	not available
cyclandelate	Cyclospasmol Cyclobral	Cyclospasmol
cyclizine	Valoid	Marzine
cyproheptadine	Periactin	Periactin
cyproterone	Androcur Cyprostat	not available

British generic name	British trade name	Australian trade name
deanol	not available	Deaner**
desipramine	Pertofran	Pertofran
dextromethorphan	Cosylan (syrup); an ingredient in several antitussive preparations	an ingredient in several antitussive preparations
dextropropoxyphene	Doloxene Distalgesic* Dolasan* etc.	Doloxene Digesic* Capadex* Paradex*
diamorphine	unbranded product only	not available
diazepam	Valium Tensium Solis Evacalm Atensine Alupram Diazemuls (injection)	Valium Ducene Pro-Pam
dichloralphenazone	Welldorm	Bonadorm**
diethylpropion	Apisate* Tenuate Dospan	Tenuate
dihydrocodeine	DF 118	Rikodeine Paracodin
dihydroergotamine mesylate	Dihydergot	Dihydergot
dihydroergotoxine mesylate	Hydergine	Hydergine
dioxyline phosphate	not available	not available
dipipanone	Diconal*	not available
dipyridamole	Persantin	Persantin Dipramol
disopyramide	Rythmodan Dirythmin	Norpace Rythmodan
disulfiram	Antabuse	Antabuse
domperidone	Motilium	Motilium
dothiepin	Prothiaden	Prothiaden
doxepin	Sinequan	Sinequan Quitaxon
droperidol	Droleptan	Droleptan

British generic name	British trade name	Australian trade name
ergotamine tartrate	Lingraine	Lingraine
	Migril*	Migral*
	Cafergot*	Cafergot*
ethosuximide	Zarontin	Zarontin
	Emeside	
fenfluramine	Ponderax	Ponderax
flupenthixol	Fluanxol	not available
flupenthixol decanoate	Depixol (injection)	not available
fluphenazine	Moditen	Anatensol
fluphenazine decanoate	Modecate (injection)	Modecate
fluphenazine enanthate	Moditen Enanthate (injection)	Anatensol Enanthate
fluspirilene	Redeptin (injection)	not available
glutethimide	Doriden	Doriden
haloperidol	Serenace	Serenace
	Haldol	
	Fortunan	
harmaline	not available	not available
imipramine	Tofranil	Tofranil
	Praminil	Melipramine
		Imiprin
		Prodepress
inositol nicotinate	Hexopal	Vasodil**
iprindole	Prondol	not available
iproniazid	Marsilid	Marsilid
isocarboxazid	Marplan	Marplan
isoxsuprine	Duvadilan	Duvadilan
labetalol	Trandate	Trandate
levodopa	Brocadopa	Larodopa
	Larodopa	Syndopa
	Berkdopa	Madopar*
	Madopar*	Sinemet*
	Sinemet*	
lithium carbonate	Camcolit	Camcolit
	Liskonum	Lithicarb
	Priadel	Manialith
	Phasal	Priadel
lorazepam	Ativan	Ativan
	Almazine	

British generic name	British trade name	Australian trade name
lormetazepam	Noctamid	not available
loxapine	not available	Loxapac**
maprotiline	Ludiomil	not available
mazindol	Teronac	Sanorex
meclofenoxate	Lucidril**	Lucidril**
medazepam	Nobrium	Raporan
meprobamate	Equanil	Equanil
	Miltown	Mepron
	Meprate	
meptazinol	Meptid (injection)	not available
methadone	Physeptone	Physeptone
methamphetamine	Methedrine**	not available
methaqualone	Melsed**	not available
	Revonal**	
methotrimeprazine	Veractil	not available
	Nozinan (injection)	
methylcellulose	Celevac	Cellulone
	Cellucon	
	Nilstim	
methylphenidate	Ritalin	Ritalin
methyprylone	Noludar	not available
methysergide	Deseril	Deseril
metiapine	not available	not available
metoclopramide	Maxolon	Maxolon
	Primperan	Primperan
	Parmid	Metamide
	Metox	
	Paramax*	
metronidazole	Flagyl	Flagyl
	Metrolyl	
	Zadstat	
mianserin	Bolvidon	Tolvon
	Norval	
midazolam	Hypnovel (injection)	not available
molindone	not available	not available
nabilone	Cesamet	not available
naftidrofuryl	Praxilene	not available
nefopam	Acupan	not available
nialamide	Niamid**	not available

British generic name	British trade name	Australian trade name
nicotine chewing gum	Nicorette	not available
nicotinic acid	unbranded product only	Nikacid
nitrazepam	Mogadon Nitrados Remnos Somnite Unisomnia	Mogadon Dormicum
nomifensine	Merital	Merital
nordiazepam	not available	not available
nortriptyline	Allegron Aventyl	Allegron Nortab
nylidrin	not available	not available
orphenadrine	Disipal	Disipal Orpadrex
oxazepam	Serenid-D	Serepax Adumbran Benzotran Murelax
oxprenolol	Trasicor Apsolox	Trasicor
oxypertine	Integrin	not available
papaverine	an ingredient in several different preparations	not available
penfluridol	not available	not available
pentifylline	not available	not available
perphenazine	Fentazin	Trilafon**
phencyclidine	not available	not available
phenelzine	Nardil	Nardil
phenmetrazine	Preludin**	not available
phenobarbitone	Luminal	unbranded product only
phentermine	Ionamin Duromine	Duromine
phenylephrine	Neophryn (nasal drops) Isopto Frin (eyedrops) Prefrin (eyedrops)	Neo-Synephrine
phenytoin	Epanutin	Dilantin
pimozide	Orap	Orap
pizotifen	Sanomigran	Sandomigran
prazepam	Centrax	not available

British generic name	British trade name	Australian trade name
prazosin	Hypovase	Minipress
prednisolone	Deltastab	Deltasolone
	Precortisyl	Prelone
	Deltalone	Deltacortef, etc
primidone	Mysoline	Mysoline
		Midone
prochlorperazine	Stemetil	Stemetil
		Compazine
procyclidine	Kemadrin	Kemadrin
promazine	Sparine	Sparine
promethazine	Phenergan	Phenergan
		Prothazine
		Meth-Zine
propranolol	Inderal	Inderal
	Berkolol	Cardinol
	Apsolol	Prolol
	Angilol	
protriptyline	Concordin	Concordin
pyridoxal phosphate	not available	not available
pyridoxine	Benadon	Pyroxin
hydrochloride	Complomant Continus	Pydox
reserpine	Serpasil	Serpasil
selegiline	Eldepryl	not available
sodium valproate	Epilim	Epilim
soya bean oil	Intralipid (injection)	Intralipid
sterculia	Prefil	Normacol
sulphinpyrazone	Anturan	Anturan
sulpiride	Dolmatil	not available
temazepam	Euhypnos	Euhypnos
	Normison	Normison
tetrabenazine	Nitoman	Nitoman
thiopentone sodium	Intraval Sodium	Intraval Sodium
	(injection)	Pentothal Sodium
thiopropazate	Dartalan	Dartalan
thioridazine	Melleril	Melleril
thiothixene	Navane**	Navane
thyroxine	Eltroxin	Thyroxinal
		Oroxine
tranylcypromine	Parnate	Parnate
trazodone	Molipaxin	not available
triazolam	Halcion	not available

British generic name	British trade name	Australian trade name
trifluoperazine	Stelazine	Stelazine Calmazine
trifluperidol	Triperidol	not available
triiodothyronine (liothyronine)	Tertroxin	Tertroxin
trimipramine	Surmontil	Surmontil
tryptophan	Optimax WV Pacitron	not available
viloxazine	Vivalan	not available
vitamin B and C	Parentrovite IM HP (injection)	Parentrovite IM HP

References

Chapter 2

1. Bleuler, E. (1911). English edition: Bleuler, E., *Textbook of Psychiatry* (Arno Press, New York, 1976).
2. Laborit, H., Huguenard, P. & Alluaume, R., 'Un nouveau stabilisateur vegetatif, le 4560 R.P', *Presse Médicale* (1952) *60*: pp. 206–208.
3. Lehman, H. E. & Hanrahan, G. E., 'Chlorpromazine, a new inhibiting agent for psychomotor excitement and manic states', *Archives of Neurology & Psychiatry* (1954) *71*: pp. 227–257.
4. Davis, J. M., 'Overview: maintenance therapy in psychiatry. I. Schizophrenia', *American Journal of Psychiatry* (1975) *132*: pp. 1237–1245.

Chapter 3

5. Wender, P. H. & Klein, D. F., *Mind, Mood & Medicine* (Farrar, Straus, Giroux, New York, 1981).
6. Morris, J. B. & Beck, A. T., 'The efficacy of antidepressant drugs', *Archives of General Psychiatry* (1974) *30*: pp. 667–674.
7. Kuhn, R., 'The treatment of depressive states with G22355 (imipramine hydrochloride)', *American Journal of Psychiatry* (1958) *115*: pp. 459–464.
8. Fox, H. H., 'The chemical attack on tuberculosis', *Transactions of the New York Academy of Sciences* (1953) *15*: pp. 234–242.
9. Delay, J. & Deniker, P., *38 cas de psychoses traitées par 4560 R.P. Compte rendu de Congres des Al. et Neurol* (Masson et Cil, Paris, 1952).
10. Ayd, F. J. jr. & Blackwell, B., *Discoveries in Biological Psychiatry* (J. B. Lippincott Co, Philadelphia, 1970).

Chapter 4

11. Priest, R. G., Amrein, U. V. & Skreta, M., *Benzodiazepines Today & Tomorrow* (MTP Press Ltd, Lancaster, 1980).

Chapter 5

12. Webster, S. G. P., 'Dementia', *Journal of Community Nursing* (1982) *1*: pp. 6–9.
13. George, C. F. & Hall, M. R. P., 'Drugs for dementia', *Prescribers Journal* (1981) *21*: pp. 272–277.

14. Coronary Drug Project Research Group, 'Long-term aspirin prophylactic therapy', *Journal of Chronic Diseases* (1976) *29*: pp. 625–642.
15. Thompson, R. A. & Green, J. R., *Stroke. Advances in Neurology Vol. 16* (Raven Press, New York, 1977).

Chapter 6

16. Oswald, I. & Adam, K., *Get A Better Night's Sleep* (Martin Dunitz Ltd, London, 1983).
17. Priest, R. G., Pletscher, A. & Ward, J., *Sleep Research* (MTP Press Ltd, Lancaster, 1979).
18. Rogers, H. J., Spector, R. G. & Trounce, J. R., *Textbook of Clinical Pharmacology* (Hodder & Stoughton, London, 1981).

Chapter 7

19. Anonymous, 'Nicotine chewing gum (Nicorette)', *Drug & Therapeutics Bulletin* (1980) pp. 83–84.
20. Musto, D. F., *The American Disease* (Yale University Press, New Haven, 1973).

Chapter 8

21. Kissell, P. & Barrucand, D., *Placebos et effet placebo en médecine* (Masson, Paris, 1964).
22. Honigfeld, G., 'Nonspecific factors in treatment: 1. Review of placebo reactions and placebo reactors', *Diseases of the Nervous System* (1964) *25*: pp. 145–156.
23. Gowdey, C. W., Hamilton, J. & Philip, R. B., 'Controlled clinical trial using placebos in normal subjects', *Canadian Medical Association Journal* (1967) *96*: pp. 1317–1322.
24. Jospe, M., *The Placebo Effect in Healing* (Lexington Books, Toronto, 1978).
25. Beecher, H. K., 'The powerful placebo', *Journal of the American Medical Association* (1955) *159*: pp. 1602–1606.
26. Benson, H. & McCallie, D. P. Jr., 'Angina pectoris and the placebo effect', *New England Journal of Medicine* (1979) *300*: pp. 1424–1429.

Chapter 10

27. Garrow, J., *Energy Balance & Obesity in Man* (Elsevier, Amsterdam, 1978).
28. Stunkark, A. J., *Obesity* (Saunders, Philadelphia, 1980).

Chapter 11

29. Harcus, A. N., Smith, R. & Whittle, B., *Pain* (Churchill Livingstone, Edinburgh, 1977).
30. Nemiah, J. C., *Physiology, Emotion & Psychosomatic Illness* (Ciba Foundation Symposium, Elsevier, Amsterdam, 1972).
31. Holmes, T. H. & Rahe, R. H., 'Stress & Breakdown', *New York Times*, June 10th, 1973.

32. Tunstall Pedoe, H., 'Epidemiology and primary prevention of coronary heart disease', *Medicine International* (1982) *1*: pp. 903–906.
33. Madders, J., *Stress and Relaxation* (Martin Dunitz Ltd, London, 1979).
34. Chaudhary, N. A. & Truelove, S. C., 'The irritable colon syndrome', *Quarterly Journal of Medicine* (1962) *31*: pp. 307–315.
35. Sutherland, J. M., Tait & Eadie, M. J., *The Epilepsies* (Churchill Livingstone, Edinburgh, 1974).
36. Shaw, K. M., Lees, A. J. & Stern, G. M., 'The impact of treatment with levodopa in Parkinson's disease', *Quarterly Journal of Medicine* (1980) *49*: pp. 283–293.

Chapter 13

37. Wuth, O., 'A method for estimating bromide concentration in blood', *Journal of the American Medical Association* (1927) *88*: pp. 2013–2015.

Useful addresses

ANXIETY AND DEPRESSION

Age Concern
Bernard Sunley House
60 Pitcairn Road
Mitcham
Surrey

Cruse (for the widowed)
126 Sheen Road
Richmond
Surrey TW9 1UR

Gingerbread (one-parent families)
Minerva Chambers
35 Wellington Street
London WC2E 7BN

Meet-a-Mum Association (self-help group)
c/o Mary Whitlock
26A Cumnor Hill
Oxford OX2 9HA

National Association for Mental Health (MIND)
22 Harley Street
London W1N 2ED

National Childbirth Trust
9 Queensborough Terrace
London W2

National Housewives Register
Antoinette Ferraro
National Organizer
245 Warwick Road
Solihull
West Midlands B92 7AH

Phobics Society
Mrs K Fisher
4 Cheltenham Road
Chorlton cum Hardy
Manchester M21 1QN

The Samaritans
17 Uxbridge Road
Slough SL1 1SN

ALCOHOLISM

Al-Anon Family Groups (UK and Eire)
61 Great Dover Street
London SE1 4YF

Alcoholics Anonymous
11 Redcliffe Gardens
London SW10 9BQ

Alcoholism Community Centres for Education, Prevention & Treatment (ACCEPT)
200 Seagrave Road
London SW6 1RQ

Aquaria
4 St Georges Street
Regent Square
Northampton

Medical Council on Alcoholism
31 Bedford Square
London WC1

DRUG DEPENDENCY/ADDICTION

Drugs Information and Advisory Services Ltd
111 Cowbridge Road East
Canton
Cardiff CF1 9AG

Institute for the Study of Drug Dependence (ISDD)
3 Blackburn Road
London NW6 1XA

Lifeline Project
Jodrell Street
Manchester M3 3HE

Release
1 Elgin Avenue
London W9 3PR

Standing Conference on Drug Abuse (SCODA)
3 Blackburn Road
London NW6 1XA

Teachers Advisory Council on Alcohol and Drug Education (TACADE)
2 Mount Street
Manchester M2 5NG

SCHIZOPHRENIA

National Schizophrenia Fellowship
78–9 Victoria Road
Surbiton
Surrey KT6 4NS

Schizophrenia Association of Great Britain
Bryn Hyfred
The Crescent
Bangor
Gwynedd LL57

MIGRAINE

British Migraine Association
178A High Road
Byfleet, Weybridge
Surrey KT14 7ED

Migraine Trust
45 Great Ormond Street
London WC1N 3HD

MISCELLANEOUS

Anorexic Aid
The Priory Centre
11 Priory Road
High Wycombe
Bucks

British Epilepsy Association
Crowthorne House
Bigshotte
New Wokingham Road
Wokingham
Berkshire RG11 3AY

Centre for the Mentally Handicapped
Sunley House
Gunthorpe Street
London E1

Dementia in the Elderly
Alzheimer Disease Society
3rd Floor
Bank Buildings
Fulham Broadway
London SW6 1EP

National Marriage Guidance Council
Herbert Gray College
Little Church Street
Rugby CV21 3AP

National Women's Aid Federation
52–4 Featherstone Street
London EC1

Parkinson's Disease Society
36 Portland Place
London W1N 3DG

Index